There's Food on Your Face

The Hippy Homemaker's

DIY Guide to

Natural Health & Beauty

Christina Anthis

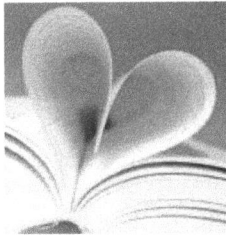

CaryPress

Table of Contents

INTRODUCTION

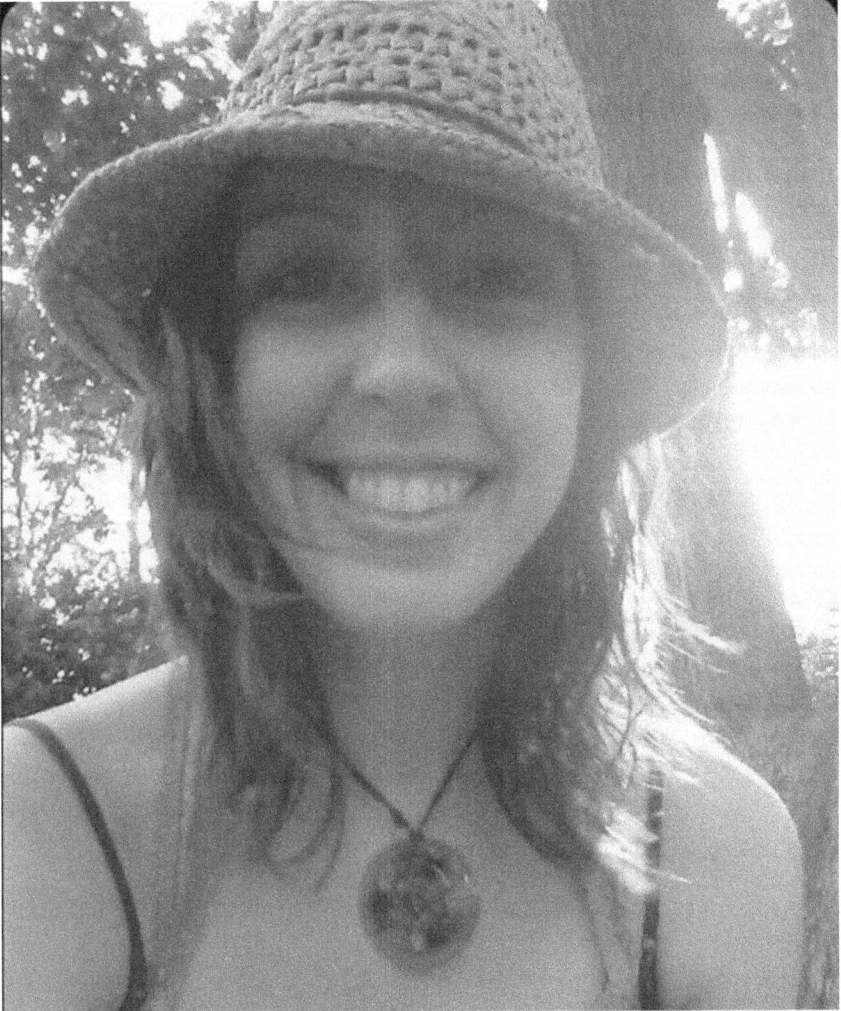

I grew up in a different world than what my son is growing up in now. In my childhood, we were fed all sorts of quick foods that hardly deserve the moniker of food. We used all sorts of products on our hair and skin that were made from synthetic ingredients and toxic chemicals. Our parents didn't know any better. We were all told that if it's approved by the FDA then it must be OK. It seemed normal to us that we didn't really know what any of the ingredients were in these products; after all, things were easier now with technology being so advanced, we didn't have to know what was in them.

The problem has never been that technology is advancing though, the problem is that with the advancement of technology, people have gotten complacent in their lives. It used to be the norm in every household for someone to bake fresh bread every other day, or to make your own deodorant, but today most people don't even realize that they have much of what they need, in their pantry and fridge, to make all of their own products and even save a ton of money in the process.

I have always been a hippy at heart. As a child I was enthralled by the rainforest and cared very deeply about the environment. I started my very first club in elementary school, called SOPA (short for Save Our Planet Association) and did everything I could to get my fellow classmates to join in on picking up trash around our local parks. As I grew up, my tree hugging ways never changed. I implemented recycling in my family's household, always looked for a more natural choice when it came to medicine, and studied environmental science in college. It never occurred to me that I needed to make a change in what I was putting into my own body and slathering all over my largest organ. I was fighting for the planet, but I wasn't fighting for myself.

When I first watched the documentary Chemerical (a documentary that discusses the toxic chemicals in our cleaning supplies, beauty products, and toiletries), I was shocked! I had no idea that all these years I had been using, breathing in, and slathering all over my skin, these products that were toxic to my health. I was aghast that this country was even allowing this to happen! I had been under the belief that that was what the FDA was there for, to keep us safe from harmful products and foods, but now I see that is clearly not the case.

This shocking revelation led me on a journey that I never could have expected. I began doing my own research and from that day forward my life has never been the same. The first thing I did was change the way that my family cleaned our house. I began learning to make my own cleaning supplies and completely changed my house over to a hippier lifestyle. I began reading and learning about nutrition, aromatherapy, herbalism, and soaking up everything that I could find on learning to do it all myself. This is how The Hippy Homemaker came to be.

I began writing my blog, The Hippy Homemaker, in June of 2012, documenting my family's conscious journey to a healthier and hippier lifestyle. As I began studying aromatherapy and herbalism, my recipes improved and my blog took off. I was suddenly thrown into a new life and was loving every minute of it.

A year later, I had written about many bath and beauty products and many of my readers were all asking for the same thing; to sell all of the products that I wrote about. I had thought that I was only on a journey to get other people to learn how to make their lives healthier by making everything for themselves, but it turned out, not everyone has the time to be able to make EVERYTHING from scratch. When I finally wizened up to this fact, I opened up my Etsy shoppe and began creating my own line of bath, beauty, and toiletries to sell to the public.

Unlike many bloggers, I tried and tested all of the recipes that I shared on my blog, and then improved upon them every time that I made them for myself. I choose to share all of my recipes for the products that I sell in my shoppe because I am still on a mission to help the world relearn how to take more initiative in their own personal care and health. For those who don't have the time, I still spend my time making natural organic products so that they too are able to have high quality products that give them the confidence in what they are putting on their bodies.

90% of body products on the market contain toxic chemicals

Did you know that your skin absorbs 60% of what is put on it? Every spray that you spray around your body, all of the cleaning supplies that you clean with, the beauty products you use daily to keep your best face forward, your bath care, your toiletries; all of these products that fill the shelves of our grocery stores contain many combinations of toxic chemicals that are known carcinogens (cancer causing). Cancer, skin allergies, infertility, birth defects, and reproductive problems have all been linked back to some of these ingredients. Next time you are shopping check the labels of your favorite products for these top toxic ingredients:

• **Parabens** – One of the most widely used preservatives in bath and beauty care products, parabens prevent the growth of bacteria, mold, and yeast in all of your beauty products. Parabens have been known to be hormone and endocrine disruptors, mimicking estrogen, and causing cancer, especially breast cancer. Parabens have even been identified in biopsy samples taken from breast and ovarian tumors. The use of parabens also has been linked to reproductive toxicity, immunotoxicity, neurotoxicity, and skin irritation.

• **Synthetic colors (FD&C Color Pigments)** – Synthetic colors that are derived from petroleum and coal tar sources, FD&C pigments are suspected to be a carcinogen, cause skin irritation, and is a known cause of ADHD in children. These synthetic colors contain heavy metal salts that deposit toxins directly into the skin. The absorption of specific colors can cause depletion of oxygen and sometimes even death.

• **Fragrances** – This category scares me the most because you really have no idea what you are getting when you see this listed on the label. A long time ago this term was created so that companies could protect their secret formulas for their specific scent creations. The problem with this is that you never know what kind of chemical concoction they've come up with to create this scent. The Environmental Working Group's 2004 analysis of potentially sensitizing ingredients in cosmetics shows that "Approximately half of all products examined list the word "fragrance" on the label. Fragrances are considered to be among the top five known allergens" They also noted that certain types of asthma attacks are "specifically triggered by, and only by, cosmetic fragrances."

• **Phthalates** – This group of chemicals is used on many of our bath and beauty products to increase the flexibility and softness of plastics. Phthalates are known to be endocrine disruptors and have been linked to breast cancer, early breast development in girls, and reproductive defects in both girls and boys. Most of the time, phthalates aren't even listed on the ingredients label. They're usually added to fragrances and become part of the "secret ingredients", therefore not having to be listed on the label at all.

• **Triclosan** – Used in many hand-soaps as an antibacterial agent, triclosan is register by the EPA as a pesticide that is considered hazardous to human heath as well as the environment. Triclosan is classified as a chemical that is suspected to be cancer causing in humans. Also known to be a hormone disruptor as well as a neurotoxin, triclosan is huge problem for the future of antibiotics. Antibiotics are a key defense against infections. When we find antibiotics in our food, bath, and beauty products our bodies begin to develop illnesses that are resistant to the antibiotics that exist on the market. With the over consumption of products containing these ingredients, we are starting to see a new generation of antibiotic resistant infections, and doctors are saying that there is nothing we can do to combat this resultant problem at this point.

• **Sodium lauryl sulfate (SLS) / Sodium laureth sulfate (SLES)** – Many of the "soaps" on the market these days (i.e. your shampoo, body wash, etc.) are not soap at all, but synthetic detergents and surfactants that are created in a lab, to clean. About 90% of the cleaning products and toiletries on the market have surfactants in them. SLS has been known to be a skin, lung, and eye irritant and most of the concern surrounding it is because of its ability to interact with other chemicals, creating carcinogens.

• **Benzoyl Peroxide** – Used in nearly every acne product on the market, benzoyl peroxide has a safety caution in its MSDS that states it is a possible tumor promoter, may act as a mutagen, and damages DNA in human and mammalians at a cellular level. Benzoyl Peroxide is also toxic by inhalation, and is a known skin, eye, and respiratory irritant.

• **Formaldehyde** – Used in many bath and beauty products in the form of preservatives called DMDM Hydantion & Urea (Imidazolidinyl). These can particularly be found in shampoos and baby soaps. These formaldehyde releasing preservatives have been known to cause joint pain, cancer, skin allergies, rashes, depression, headaches, chest pains, ear infections, and even insomnia.

• **Sunscreen Chemicals** – Many sunscreens on the market contain concerning ingredients. These chemicals are known endocrine disruptors and are easily absorbed into the body. There is increasing concern that these chemicals potentially cause damage to the skin at a cellular level, including skin cancer. Some of their common listed names on the back of your sunscreen bottle are benzophenone, PABA, avobenzone, homosalate, and ethoxycinnmate.

Health doesn't come from plastic bottles

If there is one thing that I have learned on my own personal journey, it's the importance of thinking of your health through the eyes of the **whole.** You can take medicine or use topical applications, but they only do so much to cover up the symptoms, rather than healing the **whole** body. The skin is your largest organ and the health of your skin is directly related to the health of the rest of your body. What you put into your body is reflected in your health. I have learned this lesson very well in my own health.

After making all of these changes in our lives, I began noticing how everyone else around us was still getting sick, but I was no longer getting sick monthly like I used to. Our son, Silas, didn't get any more ear infections, and our household hasn't seen an infection of any sort since before our hippy days. Back then, it seemed like pretty much everything was wrong with my health. I suffered from narcolepsy, Poly Cystic Ovarian Syndrome, Endometriosis, severe nerve pains from previous spinal cord surgeries, stomach pains, gas pains, acid reflux, light-headedness, headaches, chronic bronchitis, IBS, and pretty much any little illness that someone around me had caught I too caught. Something magical happened with each month that passed. We were getting healthier and healthier. We were feeling better. We are much happier now that we are healthier.

Making your own products saves money

If you are like most people around the world, myself included, you are not a part of the elite few who can afford to buy every awesome thing they see on the market at any price. If you are like us, your family is also trying to pinch the pennies any which way possible, just to get by. Don't fret, because you are not alone. One of the biggest perks that I have noticed in these last few years of making my own products at home, is that by making everything myself, we have saved a TON of extra money to put back into buying better food. The mark-up on many beauty items that profess to do magical things, is pretty crazy. Once you learn how to make your own beauty products and toiletries, you will begin to realize just how awesome of a product you can get for such a cheap price.

This journey to a new you will transform your life

I am so glad that you have chosen to take this journey with me. I hope that you enjoy your journey in learning to create your own natural bath and beauty products. May you be blessed with health, hippiness, and a certain kind of love for homemade gifts that are good for your mind, body, and soul!

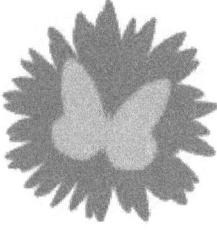

CHAPTER 1

Ingredients & Basics

With your skin being the largest organ that is a part of your body, it would make sense that what you put on it is just as important as what you put in it. The ingredients that go into your products are the most important part of the recipe. These are the magical substances that will do the job that you are creating these products to do. For the best benefit of these products, you will want to try and get as many of them organic, as possible. It defeats the purpose of avoiding toxic ingredients when the method the ingredients were created is also unhealthy. It is just as important to look at pesticides in our body care products as it is in our food. Remember...largest organ. That is all that I need to hear to remind me how important my ingredients are to my health.

Carrier Oils

Carrier oils, simplistically put, are liquid oils that are used in aromatherapy and massage to dilute essential oils and absolutes, as well as many bath and beauty products. Most essential oils should be diluted with a carrier oil so as to prevent skin irritation. All carrier oils are used for moisturizing and many have regenerative properties for both hair and skin applications. Carrier oils are widely used in lotions, creams, salves, lip balms, bath salts, facial care and more. Carrier oils, unlike essential oils, are not volatile so they will not evaporate. The best choice for carrier oils are ones that are unrefined and always cold-pressed to preserve the most amount of healing properties.

There are many carrier oils out there that are filled with amazing regenerative benefits for your hair and skin, but for the purpose of this book, I am only going to go over the most commonly used carrier oils that you will see frequently used throughout this book.

Avocado Oil – An ultra-moisturizing oil, avocado oil is used for dry hair and skin treatments, helping to soften rough skin, deeply hydrate, and refine the texture of skin. A non-comedogenic oil (pore clogging), this oil helps to refresh dry and damaged skin. Avocado oil is rich in age defying antioxidants and fatty acids. This vitamin rich herb is great in deep conditioning hair treatments, facial moisturizing serums, and winter hand creams.

Coconut Oil – This all around amazing oil is one of my favorites and pretty much used in everything that I make. Known to be antibacterial, anti-fungal, anti-inflammatory, and anti-microbial, this oil is great to use in all of your healing herbal salves, toothpastes, deodorant, and body butters. Rich in fatty acids, coconut oil makes one of the best moisturizers by itself, hands down. All of these healing properties also make coconut oil the perfect oil to use for oil-pulling (an Ayurvedic practice where you basically swish a nourishing oil around in your mouth for 20 minutes first thing in the morning to rid your body of toxins, whiten your teeth, and even see improved energy.) My favorite part of coconut oil is its light coconut smell and taste. It reminds me of a tropical beach!

Grapeseed Oil – The oil extracted from the seeds in grapes, grapeseed oil is full of antioxidants just like wine. Rich in linoleic acid, grapeseed oil is great for promoting skin health and treating acne. Grapeseed oil is an astringent oil, helping to tighten skin and close the pores. Also anti-inflammatory, grapeseed oil is great for treating wrinkles and dark under eye circles. One of the oils that is very rich in vitamin e, grapeseed oil has a longer shelf life than some of the other carrier oils.

Hemp Seed Oil – A dry emollient oil (softens the skin without leaving it too greasy), hemp oil is one of my favorite carrier oils to use. Rich in essential fatty acids and vitamin e, this oil is great for all skin types, and has been known to help relieve acne. Hemp seed oil is also a really great hair conditioner. With 25% of it protein, hemp seed oil helps to strengthen and repair cell damage within the hair. It's emollient properties help hair to maintain moisture and to stimulate hair growth. Hemp seed oil, one of the three base oils for my Foxy Face moisturizing serum, contains agents that give it anti-inflammatory properties, as well as it's natural antioxidant properties. This makes the oil not only to help clean and detoxify your skin, it also evens out your skin tone. Because it's oil doesn't stick to your skin and clog your pores like many other oils can do, it's a great way to safely moisturize your skin without leaving a greasy residue. Hemp Oil is also a great natural way to safely brave the sun's rays, and is found in many popular sunblocks.

Jojoba Oil - Pronounced "ho-ho-ba," this carrier oil is actually a liquid wax rather than an oil. Jojoba oil is extracted from the seed of the jojoba plant. It contains large amounts of the necessary vitamins and antioxidants that help improve hair, skin, and nails. One of the best oils for acne/oily skin types, jojoba oil is similar in its make up to our skin's sebum. This golden colored oil can be used to help prevent breakage in hair. It locks in moisture while securing the hair cuticle. Jojoba oil has been known to help strengthen and protect hair from heat damage, reduce frizziness,

Olive Oil – One of the most nourishing oils that is found in the majority of pantries around this country, olive oil is a multipurpose, ultra moisturizing oil. Rich in vitamins, minerals, and fatty acids, olive oil not only prevents aging in the skin, but also helps reduce the appearance of fine lines and wrinkles. Mediterranean cultures have been using olive oil in their bath and beauty routines for centuries. Rich in vitamins A and E, olive oil has been known to hydrate the skin as well as maintain it's softness and elasticity. I most commonly combine olive oil and coconut oil when making herbal oil infusions for my healing salves, though it works alone as well.

Rosehip Seed Oil - One of the most nourishing oils that you can put on your face, I use rosehip seed oil in all of my facial moisturizing serums. Many studies have been done on this oil and it's skin regeneration capabilities and each one has blown away the competition. These tests studied people with extensive facial scarring, acne scarring, deep wrinkles, UV damage, radiation damage, burn scars, surgical scars, premature aging, dermatitis, and other skin related problems. In these tests, rosehip seed oil regenerated the skin, reduced scars and wrinkles, prevented the advancement of wrinkles and aging, and helped skin to regain its natural color and tone.

Essential Oils

Essential oils are highly concentrated aromatic oils that are extracted from certain flowers, leaves, grasses, fruits, roots, and trees. These oils contains the volatile compounds from those specific plants they were extracted from, many of which are isolated for use in pharmaceutical medicine. Used in many things from beauty products, to food flavoring, to aromatherapy, essential oils are very diverse in their uses and have many impressive healing qualities. I personally use essential oils in my daily life for everything from cleaning my house to healing my sons boo boos. Since we began our journey with essential oils in our home, we have gradually become healthier, happier, and much prettier smelling. There are many great essential oils that are capable of many different healing purposes, but this book is not an aromatherapy book, so for the purpose of this book I will only lightly cover some of the uses that these essential oils have for use in the recipes you will be learning. It's extremely important that you do as much research as you can about each oil that you are using. One drop of these oils is as concentrated as 65 cups of tea of that same herb. This means that if use incorrectly, they can be dangerous. In this book I will not tell you to ingest essential oils internally and will always suggest a carrier oil for application. Do not apply essential oils neat (without carrier) to your skin, as they can cause irritation and sensitization. Certain citrus essential oils should also be used with care. Lemon, lime, bergamot (unless specified as bergaptine-free) and grapefruit can all cause a sun sensitization, resulting in blisters or a sunburn on the area of application after sun exposure. For the most current and up to date scientific information on the safety of specific essential oils, I suggest reading Robert Tisserand's "Essential Oil Safety" 2nd Edition. **SAFETY TIP:** In the event of contact with eyes or other sensitive area do NOT wash with water. **Wash affected area with a carrier oil rather than water.** Using water to try to remove the essential oil, will not rid your skin of the oil, rather it will further disperse the oil across your skin.

Chamomile – A member of the ragweed family, chamomile has been used for centuries in teas, salves, and other applications. Chamomile essential oil is such a handy essential oil for people of all ages. One of the few essential oils that are safe for babies (over 6 months of age), this sweet apple smelling oil is great at calming the mind, uplifting the mood, easing tension, and reducing inflammation. Chamomile can also be used in natural hair dyes for blonde hair and in anti-aging creams to reduce the appearance of fine lines and wrinkles.

Clove – Spicy and sweet, this essential oil is highly anti-fungal. Used for centuries in the dental world, cloves are antiseptic and great at relieving pain. I use clove essential oil in both my arnica salve and my Aunt Flo's Soothing Salve, specifically for it's warming pain-relieving abilities. During the winter time I really love to combine sweet orange essential oil with clove essential oil. It reminds me of the pomanders we used to make every year in elementary school. **NOT SAFE FOR CHILDREN UNDER THE AGE OF 2**

Eucalyptus – This essential oil is very popular and widely used in a variety of applications. It's ability to open up the chest and allow for easier breathing is one of the main reasons it's used in many vapor rub applications. Highly antibacterial and antiseptic, this essential oil is used in everything from mouthwashes to acne washes. Eucalyptus' fresh scent is refreshing and stimulating, and can help to freshen up smelly pits too! **NOT SAFE FOR USE IN CHILDREN UNDER THE AGE OF 10.**

Geranium – Highly fragrant and floral smelling, geranium essential oil has been known throughout history as a powerful wound healer. Used both in the fragrance and medicinal industry, geranium essential oil is often used in many facial creams, lotions, and many other beauty applications as well. This oil is one of the main oils in my Aunt Flo's Soothing salve for its ability to balance feminine hormones and help with the female reproductive system. It can be used to help promote stability and balance emotionally.

Lavender – One of my all-time favorite essential oils, I pretty much use lavender essential oil in everything that I do. It's all around ability to do just about anything asked of it was what made me first fall in love, but it's smell is most certainly like no other. Neither feminine nor masculine, lavender essential oil is great for use in products for all genders. Used in healing salves, lavender essential oil is antibacterial, anti-fungal, and antiseptic. Used in facial care regime's this oil is highly beneficial at rejuvenating skin cells and blemishes. Great for all skin types, lavender can be used in toners, facial cleansing grains, moisturizing serums and more! Lavender is also one few essential oils that is safe for babies (6 months of age and older). This is one of the very few essential oils that is safe to apply to skin neat without irritation. Did you know that mosquitoes hate lavender?

Lemon – Cold-pressed from the peel of lemons, lemon essential oil smells just like the fruit it is squeezed from. Used in everything from bath and beauty products to food and cleaning products, lemon essential oil is a naturally uplifting oil that is helpful in reducing scars and spots, as well as help with acne, cuts and scrapes, and more. Lemon essential oil is a natural air disinfectant and is also a natural insecticide, making it a great addition to your bug-off sprays.

Peppermint – Peppermint is most popular nowadays in our tooth care regime's here in America. This minty fresh essential oil is a well known digestive aid, but is so much more beyond that. Used in burn care for cooling, peppermint essential oil has antibacterial properties that not only numbs the pain but also helps to keep your injury clean. This "hot" oil should be used sparingly and ALWAYS with a carrier oil so as not to cause too much burning to the skin. Not only is peppermint a natural insecticide, repelling many different types of pests, but it also great at freshening up the air in your home. **NOT SAFE FOR CHILDREN UNDER THE AGE OF 6.**

Rosemary – There is much history and folklore that surrounds rosemary, both the plant and the oil. This fragrant oil has been prized for centuries for it's amazing abilities to cleanse and sterilize the air. Used in ancient hospitals, on deathbeds, and even at most weddings, this essential oil is steeped in culture and history. Used in many hair care products, rosemary is great for aiding in the regrowth and strengthening of hair. Rosemary oil also has been known to help awaken the senses, increase mental capacity, and increase memory. When used as a study aid, rosemary essential oil helps you to focus and retain more information. **NOT SAFE FOR CHILDREN UNDER THE AGE OF 8.**

Sweet Orange – One of the most used essential oils in my house for everything from cleaning and bug-killing to uplifting our moods, sweet orange essential oil is a great essential oil to have around. Cold-pressed from the peels of oranges, sweet orange essential oil has a lovely uplifting sweet scent that is known to help calm the mind and raise spirits. Commonly used in household cleaners for it's high d-limonene content, orange oil is the perfect addition to most diy cleaning recipes because it cuts grease while killing all the germs.

Tea Tree – Tea tree essential oil has strong antibacterial and antiviral properties making it a great addition to healing salves, acne products, and deodorants. Widely known for its healing properties for the skin, tea tree's anti-inflammatory and antibacterial properties make it the number one essential oil used for acne issues of all kinds. Naturally anti-fungal, tea tree essential oil is great for use in fungus salves and even for cleaning mold in your bathtub.

Thyme – Medicinally, thyme essential oil is known for its highly antiseptic and disinfectant properties, but it's also used in household cleaning supplies for this purpose as well. In ancient Greece, Thyme was used to fumigate, cleanse the air in hospitals, as well as to treat chest ailments and other upper respiratory issues. Commonly found in mouthwashes and vapor rubs, thyme essential oil is a powerhouse antiviral that freshens breath too! There is a difference between red thyme and white thyme. White thyme is safe for use in children

Butters

Cosmetic butters are simply fabulous for pampering your inner God or Goddess. These luscious melt-on-your-skin moisturizers are one of the main ingredients in many bath and beauty recipes, including salves, lotions, and creams. There are many types of butters out there that can be used in place and substitution of the butters called for in my recipes. I only use three different types of butters in this book, because they are the easiest butters to come by when shopping for ingredients locally or online. When making substitutions in recipes, it's important to know that some butters are harder than other butters and can be substituted for less if you want to keep the same consistency in the recipe. You can choose to use less beeswax instead of less butter, if the recipe calls for it.

Cocoa Butter – Pressed from the seeds of the Cacao tree, cocoa butter is a fragrant butter, smelling deliciously of chocolate. Cocoa butter is harder than Shea butter and mango butter and can sometimes be substituted for beeswax in a recipe, though it is not as hard as beeswax and will melt when it comes in contact with your skin. This butter is commonly found in most cosmetic preparations on the market and is widely used in stretch mark creams and butters.

Mango Butter – Very similar to the color and texture of cocoa butter, mango butter is an odorless white butter that is very moisturizing to your skin. Usually expeller pressed from the seed kernel of the Mango tree, mango butter is great in body butters and lotions for an exotic treat rich in fatty acids.

Shea Butter – Made from the vegetable fat of Karite tree, Shea butter is my number one choice in all of my skin care products that I make and use. Extremely good for healing all sorts of skin problems form acne to eczema, Shea butter has been known to heal all sorts of burns and wounds in record time. This butter can get gritty when it is melted and re-cooled. To prevent this, I suggest allowing the Shea butter to sit on the heat for 20 minutes before removing to add other ingredients. If your Shea butter turns gritty, never fear, it's just a texture thing. It does not harm the healing powers of your product. You can once again remelt it to fix the problem, but it's really not worth the time since the product is fine.

Hydrosols/Flower Waters

When distilleries make essential oils, they put plant material into a pot and pour water on top of the material for distilling. When the process is finished that resultant water not only has the benefits of the herbs themselves, but hydrosols also contain a tiny amount of the essential oil too. These gentle waters are much safer versions to use for babies and pets, and can replace the water in any cosmetic recipe, for an added herbal boost. It is important to be sure that your hydrosol is not cut with anything extra, as many low quality suppliers can and will cut both hydrosols and essential oils with. Most hydrosols need to be stored in the fridge for the longest shelf life. Most hydrosols have an herby or grassy smelling aroma to them, and are subtle in comparison to essential oils, but they too carry medicinal properties of the herb in them.

Clays

Clays are one of the ingredients that I always keep on hand. Filled with minerals that your skin, hair, and body need, clays are an essential ingredient to keep on hand in your home for both medicinal and beauty purposes.

Bentonite Clay - Rich in bone feeding minerals such as calcium and potassium, bentonite clay is a fabulous non-toxic teeth cleaner, facial mask, and even hair mask! Not only can you take bentonite clay internally for detoxifying purposes, but the high mineral content that this clay contains also helps to re-mineralize the teeth! NOTE: Do not house this in anything metal (including the lid) or use metal utensils when using bentonite clay. Bentonite clay is negatively charged (the reason it's able to absorb and purify toxins in the body) and when it touches metal, the positive charge deactivates some of it's amazing benefits.

French Green Clay - French green clay is high in minerals as well as decomposed plant matter (the reason French Green Clay is green!), giving your skin a large drink in mineral magic. Used extensively for its extremely absorbent powers, French Green Clay is great for use on acne/oily skin types helping to tighten pores and soak up oils.

Rhassoul Clay - Rhassoul clay is usually mined from the Atlas mountains in Morocco. It contains higher percentages of silica, magnesium, potassium, and calcium than other clays. One of the most luxurious clays, rhassoul clay is used in most high end spas around the world.

White Kaolin Clay (a.k.a. white cosmetic clay) – One of the most common and versatile clays used in cosmetic applications, white kaolin clay is in just about everything from body powders and dry shampoos to deodorant and face masks. White kaolin clay is the perfect choice for sensitive skin when other clays are too harsh.

Herbs

There are many MANY herbs we could talk about here, but for the purpose of this book, I will stick to the main ones you will see frequently throughout the book.

Black Walnut Hulls – Often used in herbal dye applications to get a deep rich brown color, this highly anti-fungal herb is also well known for its laxative abilities. The most commonly used herb in anti-fungal creams and sprays, black walnut hulls are also antibacterial, antiseptic, and anti-parasitic. Any really good herbal salve for fungal infections will have black walnut hulls in it.

Calendula – This golden flower of Sol, the Norse sun goddess, has been healing wounds for thousands of years. Also called pot marigolds or garden marigolds, calendula is well known for it's amazing ability to help heal cuts, scrapes, abrasions, acne, eczema, burns, bee stings, and more! Calendula helps to stimulate collagen at the site of the wound, helping to minimize scarring and even assist with stretch marks. When added to herbal hair dye applications, this can help with golden highlights within blonde and red tones.

Chamomile – A well-known soother as well as digestive-aid, chamomile is very gentle on the skin too, making it perfect for sensitive skin types. Chamomile contains alpha-bisabolol. This compound reportedly reduces the appearance of fine lines and wrinkles by accelerating the healing process of the skin, while also possessing anti-irritant and anti-inflammatory properties. Chamomile has been used for centuries to help calm a colicky baby.

Hibiscus – Rich in anti-aging alphahydrody acids and amino acids, hibiscus is great at reviving hair and skin and reducing inflammation. Hibiscus is known as the Botox plant because of its abilities to help lift and firm the skin. It is also high in vitamin C, making it great for use in anti-aging products. Not only does hibiscus add shine, soften, and repair your hair, it also is useful in herbal hair dye applications where you might want red tones. Hibiscus give such a lovely hue of red/pink that I even use it to make my vegan lip stain that I sell in my shoppe.

Horsetail - This astringent herb is really great for hair and bone health! Horsetail, a grassy smelling herb, is well-known in the hair care industry and used in many shampoos and conditioners because of its extremely high silica content. It helps soften and condition hair when used in tea rinses and hair masks.

Lavender – One of the most renown herbs, lavender is most famous for its relaxing effects to the mind, but it also helps to soothe skin as well. It is rich in a compound called linalol, that assists the skin in healing while also preventing tissue degeneration, keeping skin firm, and preventing wrinkles. Lavender also encourages the growth of new skin cells due to its cytophylactic properties and helps to heal wounds, scar tissue, acne, eczema and problem skin. It is anti-viral, anti-inflammatory, anti-toxic, anti-bacterial and an anti-septic.

Lemonbalm – Also known as Melissa, lemonbalm was used frequently by the Ancient Greeks and Romans medicinally for a wide variety of problems. It is well known to aid in healing skin and is great for acne/oily skin. Lemonbalm is particularly well known for treating cold sores. Lemonbalm is an astringent herb, helping to remove excess oils and to tighten the skin. It's anti-inflammatory and antibacterial properties make it great for use in both owie creams and soothing muscle salves.

Marshmallow Root – Used for centuries and even mentioned in Homer's Iliad, this skin and hair healing herb, is one of my favorites to use in herbal hair care because of the "slip" it gives to help DE-tangle your hair. Marshmallow root is filled with mucilage, making it produce a gelatinous type substance along the same terms as flax. You can use marshmallow root powder to thicken up your homemade hair conditioners and sprays.

Nettle - This wonderful herb not only is chock full of vitamins and minerals but also helps to stimulate blood flow within the scalp, aiding in hair growth and shine. Nettle has also been known to prevent dandruff and is used as a tea for seasonal allergy relief.

Peppermint – Peppermint leaf has so many uses in the home. It's great as a tea to aid in digestion and help sooth nausea. It's great in skin and hair care products because it stimulates the skin and because of its highly antiseptic nature, is great in oral health care too. Peppermint also helps to repel many rodents, spiders, and flying bugs!

Rose – The quintessential love herb, roses have been given to women all over the world as the ultimate offering to the goddess within her. Roses have such a lovely fragrant smell, and have been used for ages in the perfume industry. The use of roses in bath houses in ancient Greece and Rome was very prevalent, to perfume the waters. Roses aren't just a delight for our noses though, they also have many healing benefits in the bath and beauty world. Rich in vitamins and antioxidants, roses make great additions to any skin care application. So gentle, their use is recommended for even the most sensitive of skin. Rose can help to sooth irritated skin, and even help heal and prevent acne breakouts. This gentle beauty has many uses!

Rosemary – Rosemary has long been used for culinary, medicinal, and bath purposes. Native to the Mediterranean, this delicious herb, has many uses. In hair care, rosemary infused oil is a well known hair growth oil that helps to stimulate the scalp for healthier and stronger hair. When used in hair dye concoctions, rosemary can help with luster and shine in darker shades of hair color. In Ancient Greece and Rome, rosemary was a known purifier (thanks to its highly antiseptic and antibacterial properties) and was burned throughout hospitals and sick rooms in people's homes. It can help repel bugs and mosquitoes, congestion, stiff muscles, and even helps to boost memory and focus.

Sage – This highly antibacterial and anti-fungal herb has long been used for both culinary and medicinal purposes. Sage has been used for centuries to gargle with as a mouthwash. Not only is sage wonderful at helping to heal canker sores, but it's astringent properties also help with sore throats, gingivitis, and sore gums. Sage has been used in by many different cultures to purify and cleanse the air. When relatives fell ill, it was common to see people waving smoking bundles of rosemary and sage, to purify and cleanse the air of germs. Sage can even be very effective at darkening gray hair and is used in hair dye concoctions for darker hair.

Witch Hazel – One of the most multipurpose herbs, this astringent healing herb is most well known and used in it's distilled form. Used on everything from cuts, scrapes, and abrasions to all sorts of skin care applications. Used in facial toners, aftershaves, owie sprays, and even hair sprays, this all-around herb is highly recommended to have on hand and in your natural first-aid k

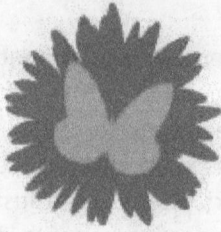

Chapter 2

Bohemi Babies

I was told that I would likely never have children when I was in my mid twenties. At first, I wasn't devastated because I hadn't thought that I wanted to have children, but as the diagnosis set in and I began to realize it was no longer my choice, I realized that I wanted kids after all. It secretly saddened me that I would not get that chance to bear my own child, but I figured at some point I could adopt a child of my own that needed a family.

Four days before I was scheduled to have another major spinal cord surgery, I felt like I needed to gain some control before the surgery came. I was freaking out inside of my head over the idea that I may not ever walk again, and knowing that I could never get pregnant, I decided I needed to take a pregnancy test. I suppose I thought that taking that test was some sort of control because I knew what it would tell me, but instead it told me that my life was about to change into a different direction than I originally thought.

I didn't get to have a choice in how I birthed my baby because of safety to my body, but I can not complain because no matter the method, I brought a beautiful healthy baby boy, Silas Thor Schreifels (a.k.a. Syfy), into this world.   Motherhood was one of the catalysts to change my lifestyle into my hippy ways. When I learned about the toxic chemicals found in many of the baby products I was using on my own baby, I was horrified that these products were even allowed to be sold on the market.

After going through my bathroom cabinets I noticed that every single item we were using in the bath, on his butt, and even on his teeth, contained ingredients that are not healthy for babies (or adults for that matter!). I was frustrated because I didn't know what was OK to buy.

The very first products that I learned how to make for my family were baby products. I was cloth diapering and cut my own microfiber wipes to have reusable wipes and stop throwing away so many baby wipes. After baby wipes, I learned to make my baby butt balm, boobie balm, and more! After making all of my baby products for a year, I began to realize I was saving a ton of money. Now, after making all of our bath and beauty products for the home for a couple years, I have noticed a drastic change in our grocery bills. That extra cash goes into buying better food and higher quality products.

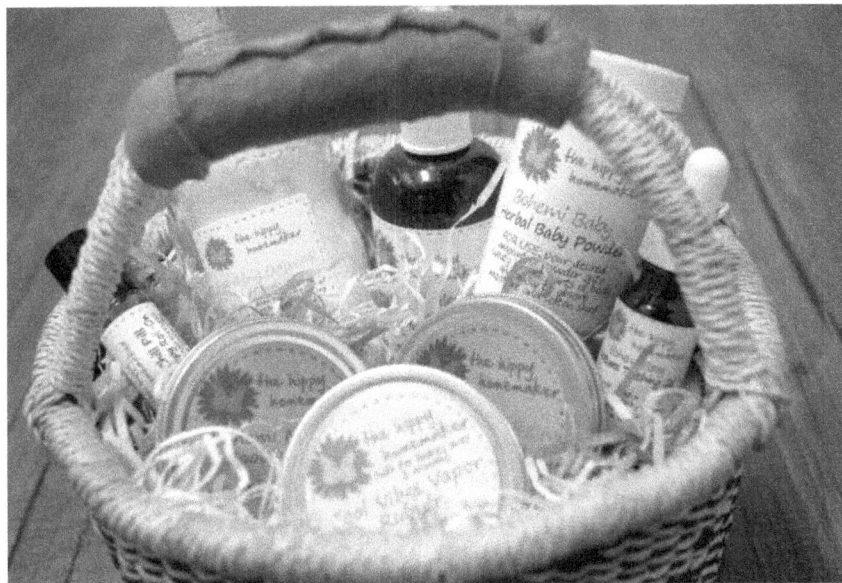

Bohemi Mama's Bloomin' Belly Butter

I make this belly butter for all of the pregnant mama's in my life! Using butters and oils that are perfect at helping minimize and reduce scarring, while softening the skin, this belly butter kept me stretch mark free during my pregnancy with Silas. I prefer to keep this butter essential oil free for the safety of pregnant mothers, but it really doesn't need any scent since the cocoa butter makes it smell of delicious chocolate, a pregnant woman's dream!

INGREDIENTS

- ¼ cup cocoa butter
- ¼ cup Shea butter
- ¼ cup coconut oil
- ¼ cup rosehip seed oil

- 1 Tbsp. Arrowroot powder
- 1 Tbsp. Vitamin E

DIRECTIONS

• Combine the butters and coconut oil in a double boiler (or makeshift one with a Pyrex/glass bowl over a pan of water) and melt.

• Once mixture has completely melted, start a timer for 20 minutes and let the butters stay at the melted temperature until the timer beeps.

• After 20 minutes, remove from heat and pour into a bowl to cool quickly in an ice bath. (larger bowl underneath filled with ice and water to help the bowl above it cool quicker.)

• In a separate smaller container, combine liquid oils, vitamin e, and arrowroot powder. It's easiest to combine the arrowroot powder into the oil with a fork.

• When it looks like the butter is half way hardened, meaning there is still a small pool of liquid on top, pour in the liquid oil/arrowroot powder concoction and take out your electric hand mixer or emulsion blender.

• I usually use the whisk attachment on my electric hand mixer, blend until there are no chunks of hardened butter left. This can not be done by hand. I usually take a spoon and chip away the bottom pieces first to make it easier to blend in the final result.

• If you added the liquid oils too soon and it's still not solid enough to pour into your containers, put the bowl of body butter mixture back onto the ice bath for a minute or two more then blend with it there in the ice bath.

• Spoon butter into the containers that you plan to store the butter in.

• The consistency of the butter will be more solidified into it's true consistency, over night.

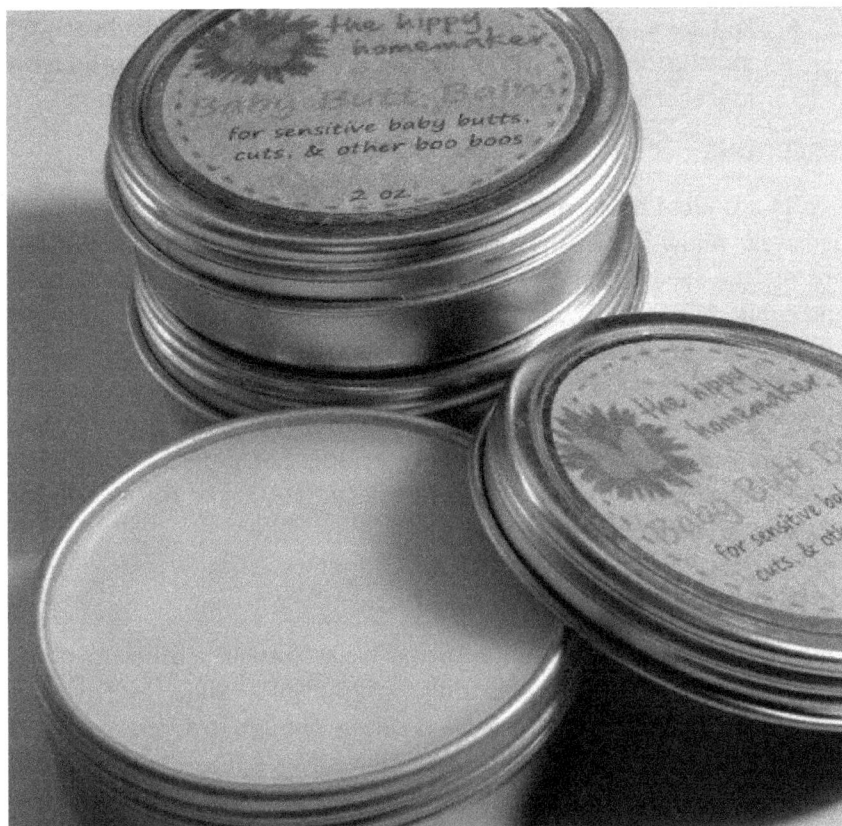

Baby Butt Balm

This recipe is cloth diaper safe and totally amazing for raw bums! You can use this on adult bums if needed too! This recipe will fill an 8 oz. Mason jar.

INGREDIENTS

- ¼ cup unrefined coconut oil

- ¼ cup extra virgin olive oil (I steep my olive oil in calendula flowers before making this salve, to add an extra herbal healing oomph to the recipe!)

- ¼ cup unrefined Shea butter

- ¼ cup beeswax pastilles

- ¼ tsp lavender essential oil

- ¼ tsp. chamomile essential oil

- ½ tsp. Vitamin e (*optional* – this not only helps heal and moisturize the skin, but also helps to give the final product a longer shelf-life by extending the life of the oils and butters.)

DIRECTIONS

• In a double boiler melt the coconut oil, olive oil, Shea butter, and beeswax. Allow your mixture to sit on the heat for 20 minutes to process the Shea butter. Shea butter is a gritty butter and when it melts and cools improperly, it can turn gritty in texture. This doesn't mean the quality of the product is bad, it's just a less appealing texture.

• Remove from heat and add essential oils and vitamin e (if using). Pour into containers to cool. Store in a cool dark place when not in use.

TO USE: Apply to a clean bum, cuts, scrapes, or burns. This salve is multidimensional for children and handy to have in the diaper bag for any kinds of unknown boo-boos.

Bohemi Mama's Boobie Balm

This healing salve was made with the breastfeeding mother in mind. With a combination of calendula infused oils, Shea butter, and chamomile essential oils, this salve is simple enough that you can put it on even before you breastfeed! Bohemi Mama's Boobie Balm will help to heal cracked and chapped nipples and to soothe and calm mama and baby.

INGREDIENTS

- ¼ cup unrefined coconut oil

- ¼ cup extra virgin olive oil

- ¼ cup beeswax pastilles

- ¼ cup Shea butter

- ¼ tsp. Roman chamomile essential oil

- ½ tsp. Vitamin e (*optional* – this not only helps heal and moisturize the skin, but also helps to give the final product a longer shelf-life by extending the life of the oils and butters.)

DIRECTIONS

• In a double boiler melt the coconut oil, olive oil, Shea butter, and beeswax. Allow your mixture to sit on the heat for 20 minutes to process the Shea butter. Shea butter is a gritty butter and when it melts and cools improperly, it can turn gritty in texture. This doesn't mean the quality of the product is bad, it's just a less appealing texture.

• Remove from heat and add essential oils and vitamin e (if using). Pour into containers to cool. Store in a cool dark place when not in use.

TO USE: Dab a small amount onto your fingers and apply generously to your breasts and nipples. Use as often as needed. A little bit goes a LONG way!

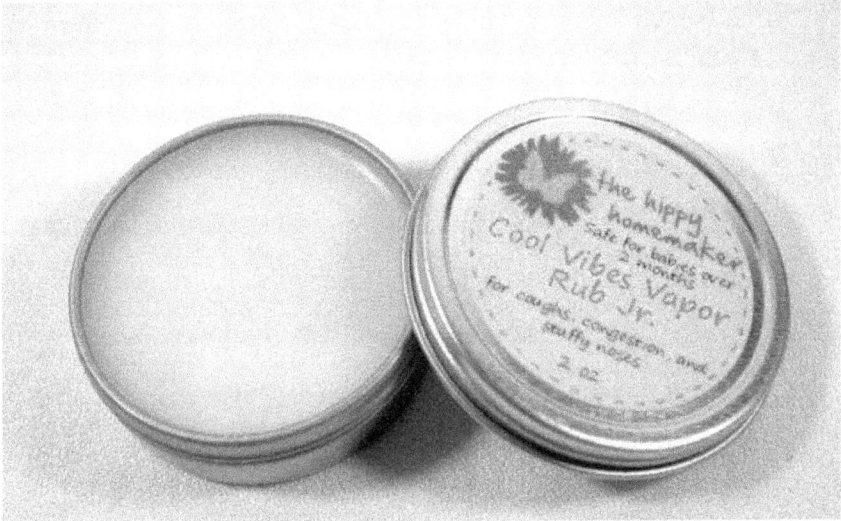

Cool Vibes Vapor Rub Jr.

Essential oils are very powerful and some are not safe for use in children, especially small children and babies. The adult version of this vapor rub contains essential oils that are not safe for use in children under the age of 10 (eucalyptus is considered safe for use in kids 10+ years, peppermint and rosemary are safe for use in children 6+ years). The menthol and cineol 1,8 content stimulates the cold receptors in the lungs and has been known to slow the breathing in young children. The fir needle essential oil in this recipe can be substituted for cypress, spruce (*picea abies, picea glauca, picea mariana, picea rubens*) or pine (*pinus divaricata, pinus resinosa, pinus strobus, pinus sylvestris*). The woodsy essential oils are all really great at helping combat congestion, coughs, and even are great expectorants! This recipe makes 8 oz. of salve. You can pour this into four 2 oz. tins or one 8 oz. mason jar, for storage. I like to make this recipe with both olive oil and coconut oil because it utilizes the natural healing benefits of both while also making the final consistency smoother. If you only have one on hand, you can replace either of the oils with the carrier oil that you have on hand.

BASE INGREDIENTS

- ½ cup extra virgin olive oil
- ¼ cup unrefined coconut oil
- ¼ cup beeswax pastilles
- ½ tsp. Vitamin e (optional, helps keeps butters and oils from going rancid longer)
- age appropriate essential oil blend

ESSENTIAL OIL BLEND 6+ MONTHS

- 30 drops fir needle essential oil (*Abies sibirica, Abies balsamea*)
- 20 drops lavender essential oil (*Lavendula angustifolia*)
- 20 drops roman chamomile essential oil (*Anthemis nobilis*)
- 25 drops sweet orange essential oil (*Citrus sinensis*)
- ESSENTIAL OIL BLEND 2+ YEARS
- 60 drops fir needle essential oil (*Abies sibirica, Abies balsamea*)
- 40 drops cypress essential oil (*Cupressus sempervires*)
- 40 drops lavender essential oil (*Lavendula angustifolia*)
- 30 drops roman chamomile essential oil (*Anthemis nobilis*)
- 25 drops thyme (*Thymus vulgaris, Thymus Zygis*)
- ESSENTIAL OIL BLEND 6+ YEARS
- 60 drops peppermint essential oil (*Mentha piperita*)
- 60 drops fir needle essential oil (*Abies sibirica, Abies balsamea*)
- 40 drops lavender essential oil (*Lavendula angustifolia*)
- 30 drops roman chamomile essential oil (*Anthemis nobilis*)
- 40 drops thyme (*Thymus vulgaris, Thymus Zygis*)

1) In a double boiler melt the coconut oil, olive oil, and beeswax.

2) Remove from heat and add age appropriate essential oil blend and vitamin e (if using). Pour into containers to cool. Store in a cool dark place when not in use.

TO USE: Dab a small amount onto your fingers and apply generously to your chest, back, and feet to help open up airways and ease breathing. You can also use a small scoop of this in a cup of hot water to make a steam inhalant. Use as often as needed. A little bit goes a LONG way! Do not rub this on your child's face or around their nose. Essential oils should be kept out of children's faces.

Herbal Healing Baby Powder

This baby powder is great because it is made with naturally healing herbs for the skin. With the help of soothing and gentle lavender and chamomile and bacteria fighting comfrey, no baby bum rash has a chance! A cheap small coffee grinder works really well to finely grind all of your herbs for any recipe requiring an herb powder, such as this one. **TIP:** If you do not have the herbs on hand, this recipe can be made with strictly the arrowroot powder and clay!

INGREDIENTS

- ½ cup arrowroot powder (this can be substituted with cornstarch but be sure it's non-GMO cornstarch!)
- ½ cup white kaolin clay (aka cosmetic clay)
- 1 Tbsp. Finely ground lavender buds
- 1 Tbsp. Finely ground chamomile
- 1 Tbsp. Finely ground comfrey
- 20 drops sweet orange essential oil

DIRECTIONS

• Combine arrowroot powder, clay, and finely ground herbs in a bowl. Add essential oils and combine. I find it is easiest to truly blend essential oils into a clay/powder if you use your fingers to thoroughly mix the powder together.
• Store in a shaker top type container.
TO USE: Sprinkle desired amount of baby powder onto a clean and dry

bum to help keep your baby's bum dry and soft.

Homemade Baby Wipes

I started out my journey as a mother to an infant, using the conventional store bought baby wipes. They seemed super handy for just about everything, but I was unaware of the nasty preservatives that are used in many of the top name brand wet wipes. I simply recycled an old plastic baby wipes container, cut several large microfiber cloths into fourths, and doused them with my baby wipes solution! These baby wipes worked great and I felt a whole lot better about what I was putting on my baby's bottom as well as into our Earth.

INGREDIENTS

- ½ Tbsp. Liquid castile soap
- ½ Tbsp. Unrefined coconut oil (you can substitute this for another oil that you might have on hand, such as olive oil)
- 1 cup water
- 2 drops lavender essential oil (*optional* – you do not need essential oils to make your own baby wipes, but they give an extra healing boost with their natural antibacterial and anti-fungal actions.
- 2 drops tea tree essential oil (*optional)*
- soft cotton cloths (1/2 of a paper towel roll if you aren't yet ready to take the plunge into wash the cloths)
- any container that will fit the solution and wipes (You can even put the solution in a spray bottle and keep the wipes dry if you so choose)
- ½ tsp. Vitamin E (*optional* – great for healing tender skin and also helps to keep the oil's shelf life longer)

DIRECTIONS

•   Combine liquid castile soap, coconut oil, water, essential oils, and vitamin E in a small bowl.

•   Arrange your wipes in your container of choice and pour your baby wipe solution all over the wipes, taking great care to get each cloth wet. I would sometimes push down into the cloths to soak up the liquid from the bottom, when I poured my solution into them.

TO USE: Use in the same way you use other wet wipes. If using reusable cloths rather than paper towels, keeping a soak bucket for the used wipes is beneficial to helping clean them in your wash.

Baby Bum Wash Spray

I originally created the Baby Bum Wash Spray as a portable version of my homemade baby wipes, that could be easily sold in my shoppe. This spray is extremely convenient and handy to have in your diaper bag! It can be used to help clean up dirty bums, messy hands, dirty faces, and more!

INGREDIENTS

- 1 tsp. Liquid castile soap
- 1 tsp. Coconut oil (you can substitute this for another oil that you might have on hand, such as olive oil)
- ½ tsp. Aloe Vera gel
- ½ tsp. Vitamin E (*optional* – great for healing tender skin and also helps to keep the oil's shelf life longer)
- distilled water to fill
- 5 drops chamomile essential oil
- 10 drops lavender essential oil
- 4 oz. PET plastic or glass spray bottle (PET plastic is the only plastic that is safe enough to use with essential oils. Glass bottles are preferred)

DIRECTIONS

- Combine all of the ingredients in a 4 oz. Spray bottle. Shake before each use.

TO USE: Spray generously on baby's bum or baby wipes, before wiping your baby's bum clean! You can spray on little hands or wipes to clean hands and faces on the go too! If by chance the coconut oil has solidified on top of the water, that means it's too cold in your house; just run the bottle under warm/hot water and shake! I use virgin unrefined coconut oil so as to utilize the amazing healing benefits that coconut oil provides!

Take a Chill Pill Calming Pillow & Room Spray

We all know those evenings, just before bed, when our baby or toddler is at their wit's end. I was at my own wit's end with the evening crazies when I developed this blend. Even now, with Silas at four and a half years old, I still use this spray daily to help us calm down and relax. You can spray this on pillows, blankets, baby clothing, bedroom, etc.

INGREDIENTS

- 1 Tbsp. Witch hazel
- 1 tsp. Aloe Vera gel (*optional* – this helps to moisturize your skin)
- 30 drops lavender essential oil
- 8 drops roman chamomile essential oil
- 15 drops tangerine essential oil
- 6 drops vanilla absolute
- water to fill
- 2 oz. Spray bottle

DIRECTIONS

• Combine ingredients in a 2 oz. Spray bottle. Shake before each use.
TO USE: Spray all over your body, pillows, clothing that needs to be refreshed before throwing into the dryer, and bed linens. Go wild! Add an aromatherapy boost to your life. I like to spray "Take a Chill Pill" on my son's feet before bed and then massage the scent into them. It always seems to help mellow him out before it's time to close his eyes.

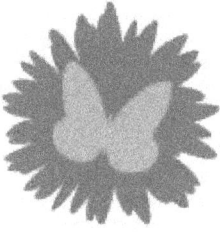

Chapter 3

Foxy Facial Care

Our faces are complicated, and finding products for them can be just as complicated with all of the harsh chemicals that can be found in many of the commercial skincare products on the market. You can easily make your own high end facial care products at home, and save hundreds of dollars. I am not kidding when I say hundreds of dollars.

I have compiled a short list of herbs and fruit powders that are great for each skin type, that can be used throughout this chapter for each of the facial care recipes. It is best if everything that you choose to use is completely dried before grinding into a powder. For citrus fruits, I utilize the dried fruit peel in my recipes. You can either harvest your own fruits/herbs/veggies, dry them yourself, and then grind them, or you can purchase them dried and ground already. For easy grinding in your own home, I suggest you purchase a cheap coffee grinder and designate it specifically for herb grinding.

Normal Skin Types – Lavender, lemonbalm, chamomile, orange peel, lemon peel, lime peel, grapefruit peel, oatstraw, horsetail, coconut flakes, pumpkin, banana, roses, hibiscus, calendula, dandelion, mango, strawberry, banana, lemon peel, lime peel, orange peel, grapefruit peel, cinnamon, clove, hibiscus, aloe, witch hazel, rosemary, basil

Acne/Oily Skin Types – Strawberry (the salicylic acid naturally found in strawberries is the main ingredient in most acne specific soap cleansers!) lemon peel, lime peel, orange peel, lemonbalm, lavender, pumpkin, cinnamon, clove, chamomile, burdock root, red clover, aloe Vera, green tea, peppermint, sage, mango, spirulina, witch hazel, feverfew, rosemary, basil, marshmallow root, licorice root, thyme, nettle, yarrow, eucalyptus, pineapple, neem leaf

Dry/Damaged/Sensitive Skin Types – Coconut flakes, coconut flour, bananas, cocoa powder, roses, lavender, horsetail, oatstraw, pumpkin, hibiscus, spirulina, mango, chamomile, calendula, aloe Vera, cocoa, pumpkin, borage, dandelion elder flower, fennel, comfrey, rosemary, avocado, cucumber, rosehips

Mature Skin Types – cocoa, coconut, roses, lavender, horsetail, oatstraw, pumpkin, spirulina, chamomile, calendula, dandelion, aloe Vera, borage, elder flower, fennel, comfrey, marshmallow root, licorice root, orange blossom, camu camu, avocado, cucumber, papaya, pineapple, rosehips

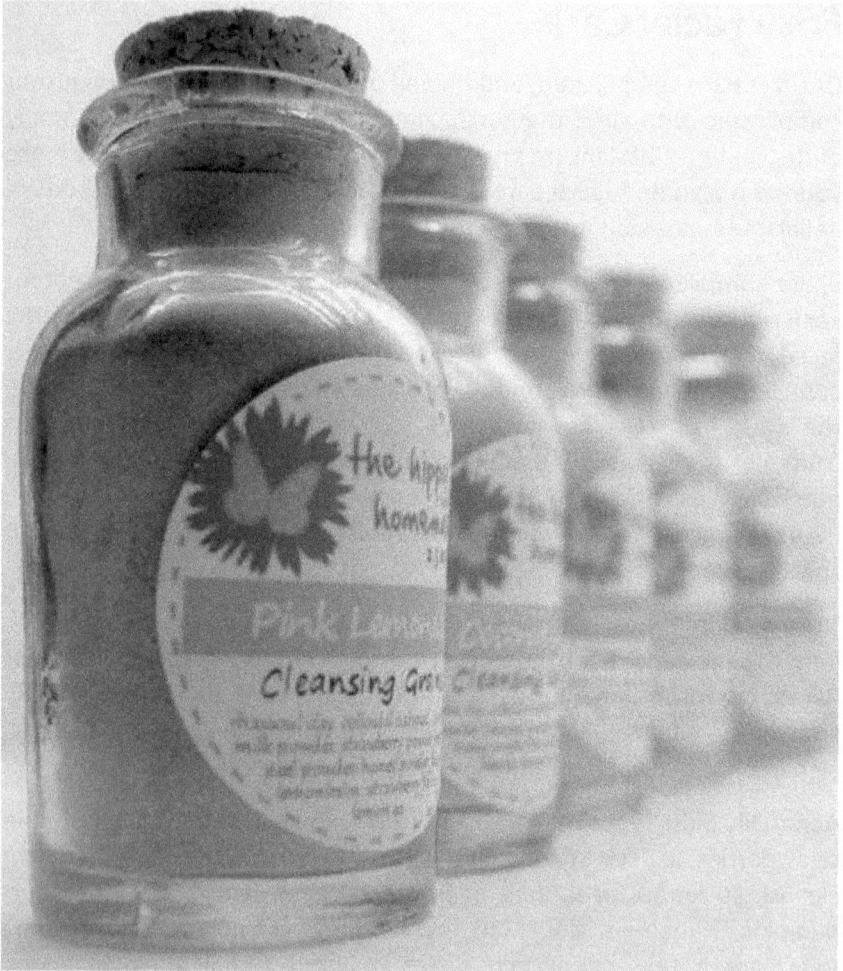

Facial Cleansing Grains

Many of my clients are so in love with my facial care set, that they buy sets for their friends to try because of their own success stories. I have tons of rave reviews talking about how nothing else was working until they switched their facial cleansing routine over to the Hippy Homemaker Foxy Facial Care Routine. I myself exclusively use my own facial care line and have never seen my skin so vibrant, clear, and beautiful. Before I created my line, I had pretty much tried every facial care line that I could fine to try and treat my acne. Nothing was working for me, even after my diet and lifestyle changes, that is until I began cleansing my face with cleansing grains.

My cleansing grains are made with only the best ingredients from nature to help smooth, soften, tighten, and firm your skin, while keeping your face blemish-free. Regular soap (if you can even call them soap) cleansers, strip your face of the important oils that keep the balance. Cleansing grains gently cleanse the skin removing dirt and dead skin cells while helping to keep the oil balance in place. This helps to heal the many different problems that people suffer from; whether it be acne, oily skin, dry skin, black heads, or rosacea (people with Rosacea should especially avoid cleansing their face with a soap cleanser, as this can aggravate and make your condition worse). I will give you two recipes, a simple basic recipe that will be much easier to adapt to your ingredients on hand, and my actual recipe for the cleansing grains that I personally sell in my shoppe.

Basic Cleansing Grains Recipe

INGREDIENTS

- 2 cups clay (white kaolin, bentonite, rhassoul, etc.)
- 1 cup finely ground oats
- ¼ cup finely ground almonds
- ¼ cup finely ground herbs (lavender, chamomile, rosemary, peppermint, sage, cinnamon in small quantities, cloves in small quantities, ginger, lemongrass, basil, and more!)

DIRECTIONS

Combine ingredients in a bowl and mix until fully combined. Store in a glass jar. As long as you avoid getting water into the jar, these cleansing grains have a really long shelf life.

TO USE: Twice daily combine 1/2 - 1 tsp. of cleansing grains with a small amount of water or hydrosol, in the palm of your hand. For an extra treat, you can use herbal tea, honey, yogurt, milk, or even fresh squeezed juice, instead of water. Apply to face, and gently scrub in a circular motion, with your fingertips in the same manner you did with your old soap cleansers. Rinse with warm water and follow with a toner and moisturizer for best results.

The Hippy Homemaker's Cleansing Grains

There are many variations that can be done with this recipe. You can choose dried fruit powders and/or herb powders that have the healing benefits for your personal skin type and from there craft your own facial cleanser that is made just for you! These make great holiday and birthday gifts too!

INGREDIENTS

- ½ cup clay (rhassoul, white kaolin, bentonite)
- ¼ cup finely ground oatmeal
- 6 Tbsp. Herb/Fruit powder (depending on which cleansing grains you want to make. If making more than one flavor, then divide the Tbsp. up. For example, the Rose & Lavender Cleansing Grains that I make in my shoppe, gets 3 Tbsp. finely ground lavender and 3 Tbsp. finely ground rose petals.)
- 1 Tbsp. Honey powder
- 1 Tbsp. Coconut milk powder
- 1 Tbsp. Flax powder
- 1-2 Tbsp. Finely ground herb for skin type

DIRECTIONS

• Combine ingredients in a bowl and mix until fully combined. Store in a glass jar. As long as you avoid getting water into the jar, these cleansing grains have a really long shelf life.

TO USE: Twice daily combine 1/2 - 1 tsp. of cleansing grains with a small amount of water or hydrosol, in the palm of your hand. For an extra treat, you can use herbal tea, honey, yogurt, milk, or even fresh squeezed juice, instead of water. Apply to face, and gently scrub in a circular motion, with your fingertips in the same manner you did with your old soap cleansers. Rinse with warm water and follow with a toner and moisturizer for best results.

Hippy Chic Face Masks

My girlfriend's and I love to celebrate the weekend with Mudmask and

Mimosa Fridays. It really puts the "Thank Goodness" back into Fridays! This weekly practice has helped us to remember to do our weekly mud masks to help smooth, soften, tighten, and firm our skin. Using a face mask once a week can really help to minimize your pores and reduce blackheads.

Making a face mask can be as easy as mashing up or pureeing fresh ingredients from your fridge. Most of the fruits, veggies, and herbs that you have on hand can be mashed up into a vitamin packed face mask. These quick and easy face masks are great for sleepovers and family bonding time too!

Refrigerator Face masks

Some of the best face masks come from ingredients that can be found in your fridge and pantry. All of the raw fruit and vegetable ingredients that you have on hand, are filled with a ton vitamins, minerals, and antioxidants to help with a whole range of facial skin care needs. Many of these ingredients are great for just about all skin types. I love to make these Refrigerator Face masks for sleepovers and with kids! You can get a good laugh out of the whole family walking around with mashed avocados on their faces.

INGREDIENTS (choose any of the following)

- Strawberries – contains vitamin C, salicylic acid (the main ingredient in acne cleansers), antioxidants and exfoliants. Salicylic acid removes dead cells from the face while tightening the pores.
- Bananas – contain vitamin C and are fabulous at helping out dry damaged skin. Bananas also give the face a natural glow.
- Mangos – rich in vitamin A (beta-carotene), contains powerful anti-oxidants, helps with skin cell regeneration, restores the elasticity of skin, helps to moisturize dry skin, prevents wrinkle formation, and helps to shield skin from clogged pores and sun damages.
- Blueberries – contains high amounts of vitamin A and C as well as antioxidants. Considered one of the miracle fruits for wrinkles, blemishes, pimples, and uneven skin tone.
- Avocados – contain high amounts of vitamin A, E, C, and K making this a miracle fruit for all face types. It's ultra moisturizing properties are great for dry damaged skin.
- Pumpkin – great for all skin types because of it's high content of vitamins A and C, but especially great for dry skin. Due to high

enzyme content, pumpkin is highly effective at hydrating, soothing, and softening excessively dry skin.

- Potato – slices of raw potato on your eyes for 15-20 minutes help with dark circles under the eyes. Masks made with peeled and blended potato can help ward off wrinkles and reduce dark spots.
- Carrot – another vegetable packed with beta-carotene, this vegetable is AMAZING at helping all face types and reducing sun damage. Carrots are great at toning and clarifying the skin and are naturally antiseptic.
- Cucumber – containing a high amount of ascorbic acid, cucumbers are really great at reducing puffy eyes and dark circles. When applied as a face mask in combination with a few drops of lemon juice, cucumbers have been known to help fade freckles and improve complexion. They also tone and tighten pores, and can help treat a sunburn.
- Other Face Nourishing Refrigerator/Pantry Ingredients – yogurt, raw unfiltered honey, aloe Vera, coconut milk, raw unfiltered apple cider vinegar, almond milk, whole milk, sour cream, cinnamon, cloves, ginger, nutmeg, sage, thyme, basil, rosemary, peppermint, eggs, nourishing carrier oil (grapeseed, rosehip seed, hemp seed, avocado seed, almond oil, etc.), gelatin, sugar

DIRECTIONS

- Choose one or more ingredients that you have available in your fridge and pantry. Blend and/or mash them into a paste.

TO USE: Apply to your face, avoiding the eyes, eye brows, and lips. Allow to sit on your face for 15-20 minutes, then rinse clean. Follow with a toner and moisturizer for best results.

Hippy Chic Herbal Face Mask Base Recipe

The masks that I make in my shoppe, sell really well! It is easy to make your own masks just like the ones that I sell in my shoppe! All you need is a base recipe and use the herbs that you have on hand. When creating a face mask specifically for your skin type, use the guide at the beginning of this chapter, to pick out the right additions for your skin type.

INGREDEINTS

- ¼ cup clay (French green clay, Rhassoul, Bentonite, white kaolin clay)

- 1 Tbsp. Finely ground oatmeal(*optional* - but adds additional healing and softening properties to the skin.)
- 1 Tbsp. milk powder or coconut milk powder (*optional* -but adds extra oomph to softness of your skin.)
- 2-4 Tbsp. finely ground herbs (*optional* - Different herbs offer different healing properties to them. In my Hippy Chic Herbal Clay Masks I like to mix it up and use more than one herb here, depending on my end goal.)
- 10-15 drops of essential oil (depending on the solo or combination of essential oils that you use. If just using one essential oil such as lavender, 10 drops will suffice. Make sure to research which essential oils you decide to put in your mask. Some essential oils, if used in excess, can cause the sensitive face some irritation or sensitization. Lavender, chamomile, and tea tree essential oils are pretty much useful for all skin types)

DIRECTIONS

•   Combine ingredients in a bowl. Mix together until completely combined. I find that it is easiest to work essential oils into the clay by using my fingers. Store in a cool dry location when not in use.

TO USE: Combine 1-2 tsp. of the mud mask with 1-2 tsp. water or hydrosol. For an extra treat, you can use herbal tea, honey, yogurt, milk, or even fresh squeezed juice, instead of water. Apply to face, neck, or any other part of the body that needs exfoliation, skin tightening, and nourishment. Allow mud mask to sit 15-20 minutes, or until hard and cracking, and rinse clean. If you want to feel the full effects of the herbs that are ground by hand for this clay mask, use hot water instead of cold, and allow the mud mixture to sit 5-10 minutes to "steep", before using.

Dancing Sunrise Hippy Chic Facemask (*for normal skin types*)

This mask is a favorite in my shoppe! It's great for pretty much all skin type and smells like a juicy grapefruit in the morning!

INGREDEINTS

- 3 Tbsp. Rhassoul Clay
- 1 Tbsp. Bentonite clay
- 1 Tbsp. Honey powder

- 1 Tbsp. Finely ground oatmeal
- 1 Tbsp. Coconut milk powder
- 1 Tbsp. Finely ground lavender buds
- 1 Tbsp. Finely ground green tea
- 20 drops grapefruit essential oil
- 10 drops lavender essential oil

DIRECTIONS

• Combine ingredients in a bowl. Mix together until completely combined. I find that it is easiest to work essential oils into the clay by using my fingers. Store in a cool dry location when not in use.

TO USE: Combine 1-2 tsp. of the mud mask with 1-2 tsp. water or hydrosol. For an extra treat, you can use herbal tea, honey, yogurt, milk, or even fresh squeezed juice, instead of water. Apply to face, neck, or any other part of the body that needs exfoliation, skin tightening, and nourishment. Allow mud mask to sit 15-20 minutes, or until hard and cracking, and rinse clean. If you want to feel the full effects of the herbs that are ground by hand for this clay mask, use hot water instead of cold, and allow the mud mixture to sit 5-10 minutes to "steep", before using.

Lavender Fields Hippy Chic Face Mask *(for sensitive skin)*

Those with sensitive faces tend to get itchy red faces when using face masks that are formulated for normal or acne/oily skin types. The key to a sensitive facemask is using white kaolin clay instead of bentonite or rhassoul! White kaolin clay is extremely gentle and will not irritate sensitive skin.

INGREDIENTS

- ¼ cup white kaolin clay
- 1 Tbsp. Honey powder
- 1 Tbsp. Finely ground oatmeal
- 1 Tbsp. Coconut milk powder
- 2 Tbsp. Finely ground lavender buds
- 1 Tbsp. Finely ground calendula flowers
- 25 drops lavender essential oil

DIRECTIONS

• Combine ingredients in a bowl. Mix together until completely combined. I find that it is easiest to work essential oils into the clay by using my fingers. Store in a cool dry location when not in use.

TO USE: Combine 1-2 tsp. of the mud mask with 1-2 tsp. water or hydrosol. For an extra treat, you can use herbal tea, honey, yogurt, milk, or even fresh squeezed juice, instead of water. Apply to face, neck, or any other part of the body that needs exfoliation, skin tightening, and nourishment. Allow mud mask to sit 15-20 minutes, or until hard and cracking, and rinse clean. If you want to feel the full effects of the herbs that are ground by hand for this clay mask, use hot water instead of cold, and allow the mud mixture to sit 5-10 minutes to "steep", before using.

Fountain of Youth Hippy Chic Facemask *(for mature/aging skin)*

This is by far my favorite facemask to use! I love the cooling feeling that I get from it and it really helps my skin look firmer, softer, and younger! This is my choice of mask for Mudmask and Mimosa Fridays.

INGREDIENTS

• ¼ cup rhassoul clay
• 1 Tbsp. Honey powder
• 1 Tbsp. Finely ground oatmeal
• 1 Tbsp. Coconut milk powder
• 1 Tbsp. Finely ground lavender buds
• 1 Tbsp. Finely ground green tea
• 1 Tbsp. Finely ground calendula flowers
• 1 Tbsp. Finely ground chamomile
• 1 tsp. Camu camu powder
• 3 drops frankincense essential oil
• 10 drops lavender essential oil
• 5 drops lime peel essential oil

DIRECTIONS

• Combine ingredients in a bowl. Mix together until completely combined. I find that it is easiest to work essential oils into the clay by using my fingers. Store in a cool dry location when not in use.

TO USE: Combine 1-2 tsp. of the mud mask with 1-2 tsp. water or hydrosol. For an extra treat, you can use herbal tea, honey, yogurt, milk, or even fresh squeezed juice, instead of water. Apply to face, neck, or any other part of the body that needs exfoliation, skin tightening, and nourishment. Allow mud mask to sit 15-20 minutes, or until hard and cracking, and rinse clean. If you want to feel the full effects of the herbs that are ground by hand for this clay mask, use hot water instead of cold, and allow the mud mixture to sit 5-10 minutes to "steep", before using.

Acne Attack Hippy Chic Facemask *(for acne/oily skin types)*

This mask is made specifically for those with acne/oily skin. Made with French green clay, it's high in minerals as well as decomposed plant matter (the reason French Green Clay is green!), giving your skin a large drink in mineral magic. This face mask is filled with ingredients that are well known to help acne/oily skin types.

INGREDIENTS

- 4 Tbsp. French Green Clay
- 1 Tbsp. Honey powder
- 1 Tbsp. Coconut milk powder
- 1 Tbsp. Finely ground chamomile
- 1 Tbsp. Finely ground lavender buds
- 1 Tbsp. Finely ground green tea
- ¼ tsp. Cinnamon powder
- 1 Tbsp. Finely ground neem leaf powder
- 1 Tbsp. Finely ground oatmeal
- 10 drops tea tree essential oil
- 2 drops lemongrass essential oil
- 5 drops lavender essential oil
- 5 drops lemon essential oil

DIRECTIONS

• Combine ingredients in a bowl. Mix together until completely combined. I find that it is easiest to work essential oils into the clay by using my fingers. Store in a cool dry location when not in use.

TO USE: Combine 1-2 tsp. of the mud mask with 1-2 tsp. water or hydrosol. For an extra treat, you can use herbal tea, honey, yogurt, milk, or even fresh squeezed juice, instead of water. Apply to face, neck, or any other part of the body that needs exfoliation, skin tightening, and nourishment. Allow mud mask to sit 15-20 minutes, or until hard and cracking, and rinse clean. If you want to feel the full effects of the herbs that are ground by hand for this clay mask, use hot water instead of cold, and allow the mud mixture to sit 5-10 minutes to "steep", before using.

Facial Toners

I love to talk a lot about using a three-step process for the daily cleansing of my face. Many people skip the most important step in facial cleansing, step 2, toning. Did you know that if you do not use a toner after cleansing your face, you are leaving your pores open to suck back in all of the dirt and grime that is around you? One of the most important steps to clean and clear skin is most often overlooked in many people's daily skin care routine. The use of a toner after cleansing your skin will help to close all of the pores that you opened during cleansing, and to balance and regulate the pH of your skin. This will help keep your oil glands from over producing oils after cleansing.

Though the witch hazel portion of this recipe can be replaced with apple cider vinegar, I have personally found that both my client's faces and my face had more problems with breaking out when I utilized apple cider vinegar. When I changed my recipe BACK to the witch hazel, all of our faces began to clear up again. I have read many stories on the internet about the use of apple cider vinegar in facial toners, but I have not personally seen any benefit from using it on myself. Try it out for a week or two and see if there is any difference in your face. You never know, it might just be the right thing for your skin.

The recipes that I am about to share with you, are the recipes that I use in my own shoppe. These toners are amazing at locking in moisture while toning the face. My clients all agree that these toners are face changing! You can make this recipe just bare bones without any of the "optional" items, and still get a very effective toner.

Moisturizing Facial Toner

BASE INGREDEINTS

- 4 oz. Spray bottle

- ¼ cup witch hazel
- 2 tsp. Aloe Vera gel (*optional* – Aloe Vera has a close pH to that of our skin's sebum, so it makes a great base for a pH balancing facial toner! Not only does it balance the pH but it also is super moisturizing too!)
- 1 tsp. Vegetable glycerin (*optional* – I use vegetable glycerin in all of my facial toners because of its natural ability to help the skin hold in moisture.)
- ½ tsp. Colloidal silver (*optional* – Colloidal silver has long been known as a natural antibiotic and is used in many veterinarian offices to help animals skin heal. Colloidal silver has also been used for treating major burns in burn units.)
- water or hydrosol to fill (I use hydrosol to fill because they add the extra herbal healing benefit to the recipe. Choose your hydrosol based on herbs for your face type, at the beginning of this chapter.)

ACNE/OILY SKIN TYPES

- 10 drops lavender essential oil
- 6 drops lemongrass essential oil
- 6 drops lemon essential oil
- 10 drops tea tree essential oil

NORMAL SKIN TYPES

- 10 drops lavender essential oil
- 6 drops cedarwood essential oil
- 10 drops grapefruit essential oil

DRY/DAMAGED SKIN TYPES

- 6 drops roman chamomile essential oil
- 4 drops cedarwood essential oil
- 2 drops ylang ylang essential oil
- 10 drops sweet orange essential oil

MATURE SKIN TYPES

- 4 drops frankincense essential oil
- 10 drops lemon essential oil
- 6 drops roman chamomile essential oil
- 4 drops geranium essential oil

DIRECTIONS

- Combine ingredients in your 4 oz. spray bottle. Shake well before each use. Store in a cool dark location such as your bathroom cabinet.

TO USE: Second step in the facial cleansing process, spray onto clean dry and face, after cleansing. Let air dry or pat gently into skin. Follow with a moisturizer.

Foxy Face Moisturizing Facial Serum

The third and extremely important step in the facial cleansing process is moisturization. When you wash your face, you cleanse it of all the old and dirty oil that has built up on it. By re-balancing your oil levels on your face, you are not only adding moisture to your face but you are preventing over production of oils as well. When your face is too dry it will go into overproduction mode and the balance gets thrown off completely.

I created this moisturizing serum with your delicate face in mind. Not only does it do an amazing job moisturizing the face, it is created with specific carrier oils and essential oils to fit the needs of your face's skin type; all while helping to reduce fine lines, wrinkles, age spots, and blemishes. The secret to Foxy Face is the two main base oils that I use for each of the skin types:

Hemp seed oil – Hemp seed oil contains agents that give it anti-inflammatory properties, as well as it's natural antioxidant properties. This helps the oil not only to help clean and detoxify your skin, it also evens out your skin tone. This oil doesn't stick to your skin and clog your pores like many other oils can, it's a great way to safely moisturize your skin without leaving a greasy residue. Hemp Oil is also a great natural way to safely brave the sun's rays, and is found in many popular sunblocks.

Rosehip Seed Oil - One of the most nourishing oils that you can put on your face, many studies have been done on this oil and it's skin regeneration capabilities and each one has blown away the competition. These tests studied people with extensive facial scarring, acne scarring, deep wrinkles, UV damage, radiation damage, burn scars, surgical scars, premature aging, dermatitis, and other skin related problems. In these tests, rosehip seed oil regenerated the skin, reduced scars and wrinkles, prevented the advancement of wrinkles and aging, and helped skin to regain its natural color and tone.

ACNE/OILY SKIN TYPES

- ½ Tbsp. Hemp seed oil
- ½ Tbsp. Rosehip seed oil
- ½ Tbsp. Jojoba oil
- ½ Tbsp. Grapeseed oil
- 2 drops lemongrass essential oil
- 3 drops tea tree essential oil
- 3 drops lavender essential oil

DRY/DAMAGED SKIN TYPES

- ½ Tbsp. Hemp seed oil
- ½ Tbsp. Rosehip seed oil
- ½ Tbsp. Avocado seed oil
- ½ Tbsp. Pumpkin seed oil
- 2 drops chamomile essential oil
- 3 drops carrot seed essential oil
- 3 drops frankincense essential oil

NORMAL SKIN TYPES

- ½ Tbsp. Hemp seed oil
- ½ Tbsp. Rosehip seed oil
- ½ Tbsp. Almond oil
- ½ Tbsp. Pumpkin seed oil
- 3 drops carrot seed essential oil
- 6 drops lavender essential oil

DIRECTIONS

• Combine ingredients in a 1 oz. glass bottle with dropper or 1 oz. Lotion pump bottle.

TO USE: Gently shake the bottle before every use, to mix all oils together evenly. Dispense 1-2 drops of oil onto the palm of your hand, rub hands together, and massage onto your face. I personally use one drop of oil for my morning application and 2 drops of oil for my evening application.

Zippy Zit Zapper Acne Spot Treatment Roll-On

Acne can be so troublesome, popping up when we least want it around.

This blemish control serum was created as a spot treatment. Zippy Zit Zapper was designed with specific carrier oils, witch hazel, and essential oils that are beneficial to skin with blemish problems. I use this recipe with a 1/3 oz. Roll-on bottle. This recipe is formulated for that size bottle. The bottle makes for easy application and storage for this spot treatment roll-on.

INGREDEINTS

- 15 drops tea tree essential oil
- 15 drops lavender essential oil
- 5 drops roman chamomile essential oil
- 2 drops carrot seed essential oil
- 1 drops lemongrass essential oil
- 3 drops cypress essential oil
- 75 drops carrier oil (I use "dry" carrier oils that are known to work well for acne. My recipe uses 25 drops each of hemp seed oil, rosehip seed oil, and grapeseed oil)
- witch hazel to fill
- 1/3 oz. Roll-on bottle

DIRECTIONS

• Combine ingredients in a 1/3 oz. Roll-on bottle, cap and store in a cool dark place, such as your bathroom drawer or cabinet.

TO USE: Shake well before use, the witch hazel and oils do not blend otherwise. Apply to affected areas up to 3x a day, especially before bed. Be sure to clean and tone face prior to application, for best results.

Easy DIY Pore Strips

I don't know about you, but I have always had a gross love for using pore strips on my nose, and then of course looking at your findings on the strip. When I made the transition to a more natural lifestyle, my beloved pore strips were one of the many casualties that sparked the need for me to create a recipe for my own pore strips.

This recipe is extremely easy and contains only two ingredients that can be found in many pantries.

INGREDEINTS

- 1 Tbsp. Organic grass-fed gelatin (*Vegan Option* – Use agar agar powder instead of gelatin!)
- 1 ½ Tbsp. Coconut milk, hydrosol, witch hazel, or water (Depending on what liquids you have on hand, you can substitute any of these option in, or even fresh pressed juice, aloe juice, and more!)

DIRECTIONS

•   Heat liquid in a small pan over medium low heat. Slowly stir in gelatin until dissolved. Allow mixture to cool just enough to be able to safely apply to skin.

TO USE: Apply with a spoon or fingers, to skin, making a thin layer on your face. Avoid using on or near facial hair and eyes. Allow to dry, and then pull off of skin, removing

Night Cream & Eye Cream

Though I absolutely love my Foxy Face Moisturizing Facial Serum for daily use, as I am now nearing 31 years old, I am beginning to think about night creams and eye creams to keep those wrinkles at bay.

You really don't need to spend $100 for a really amazing night cream! I came up with this recipe, after I saw the prices for many of the great organic night creams and eye creams on the store shelves.

The Hippy Homemaker's Magic Night Cream

This night cream is simply AMAZING. I am not kidding. Every single time that I have made this for my friends, family, and clients, I hear about how super soft their skin has become. I can't help but touch my face a lot, after using this night cream regularly, because I am always so in awe of how soft my skin has become. This recipe makes enough 1 oz. batches, that you can share this with your friends and family, and become their favorite person!

INGREDEINTS

- 2 Tbsp. Witch hazel
- 2 Tbsp. Aloe Vera gel
- ¼ cup distilled water (It is important to use distilled water so that your cream will have a longer shelf life. If you do not have

that on hand, filtered water is your next best bet, but still may have bacteria in it.)

- 2 Tbsp. Shea butter
- 1 ½ Tbsp. Emulsifying wax
- ½ cup liquid oil (I use rosehip seed oil, hemp seed oil, and pumpkin seed oil, but you can can use any combination of carrier oil that you have on hand.)
- 1 tsp. Vitamin e (*optional* - great for healing skin and also helps to keep the oil's shelf life longer)
- 10 drops frankincense essential oil
- 20 drops lavender essential oil
- 5 drops lemon essential oil
- 5 drops carrot seed essential oil
- 10 drops roman chamomile essential oil

DIRECTIONS

•   In a double boiler, heat Shea butter, emulsifying wax, and carrier oil until melted. Allow mixture to sit on the heat for 20 minutes, to process the Shea butter.

•   While the oil/butter mix is processing, in a separate small pan, heat witch hazel, aloe Vera gel, and distilled water over medium/low heat.

•   Remove both mixtures from heat and allow to cool 5 minutes or when both mixtures are the same temperature.

•   Pour water mixture into a medium sized mixing bowl (or a blender depending on what you have to mix with. You can do this in the blender instead of with a hand mixer). While blending water mixture with a hand mixer, slowly pour oil/butter mixture into water mixture.

•   Once emulsified (meaning mixture is blended together without oil and water separating), you can mix in the essential oils and vitamin e if using either. This recipe can be made without the essential oils if you do not have them on hand. It will still seriously moisturize your skin with or without the essential oils.

•   Store in a glass container in a cool dark location. Keeping this in the fridge will more than double the shelf-life.

TO USE: Using a small dab of cream, massage very lightly into skin. This cream is best use at night before bed, though it is light enough that you can use it in the morning too if you need to.

Soothing Cucumber Eye Treatment

Cucumbers have long been used in helping reduce swollen under eye "bags". They help with moisture and are very soothing and calming to the skin. You can just slice a cucumber and apply the slices to your eyes, while resting, but this eye treatment is even more effective! You can also use this treatment as your face's moisturizer. It's fabulous at reducing redness, itchy irritation, and really helps dry skin recover quickly.

INGREDEINTS

- 1 medium sized cucumber, peeled, seeded, and cubed.
- 2 Tbsp. Aloe Vera gel (you can substitute water for this, but of course the aloe is the better option for maximum moisture and reduction of inflammation.)

DIRECTIONS

• Combine ingredients in a blender or food processor and blend until a thick, juicy pulp is created.

• Pour cucumber mixture through a strainer, catching the juice in a bowl. Store the juice in the fridge for up to 3 days.

TO USE: Using a cotton cleansing pad or cotton ball, apply cucumber treatment around the eyes and all over face if desired.

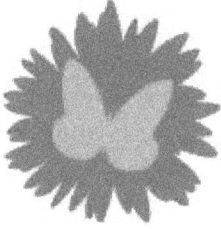

Chapter 4

Natural Body Care

One of the things I love the most about making my own body care products, is how much money I save for such high quality products! Over the course of a year, we shell out thousands of dollars for all of our body care products, and possibly more than that depending on how good of quality those products are. To top it off, most of the products you find at your local market, contain toxic ingredients that are absorbed into our skin and enter our bloodstream.

I began making my own body care products because of these suspect ingredients. I feel a tremendous amount of satisfaction knowing exactly what is in the products that my family uses. The best part about these body care recipes, is that everyone you know needs something from this chapter, which makes them fabulous gifts during the holidays or for birthdays! I like to customize these recipes to people's likes and needs to make it even more special!

Luxurious Whipped Body Butter

Body butter has to be the greatest thing since sliced bread. Seriously, before I had first learned to make body butter for myself, I had only ever used lotion. That first time that I slathered on my own body butter concoction and felt just how soft and smooth it made my skin, I never wanted to go back. My skin has never felt softer, and happier with me than after I put on fresh homemade body butter.

The best part is, this makes a really great holiday gift. Whether you scent it with essential oils or leave it plain with the nutty scent of the butters, everyone out there could use a good moisturizing body butter during the winter. You can put this butter into a really cute glass jar such as a mason jar, decorate it and fill all the stockings in the house with it.

Body butter is made with oils and butters, not water

The truth is, not only is it really easy to make, it is so much more moisturizing than lotion because it's not made with water. Being made with only oils and butters also means that there is no need to worry about preservatives either. Anything made with water needs a preservative to prevent bacteria from growing. Water also makes it where it sinks into the skin immediately so you get immediate moisture with a lotion but not an all day moisture. With body butters, the moisture is super healing to the skin because it keeps the skin hydrated for a much longer period of time.

There is a secret to silky smooth body butter

What a lot of authors out there fail to mention, when it comes to making your own body butter, there is actually a secret to melting the butters so that they don't get grainy later. When I started making body butters for my shoppe on Etsy, I sold body butters that I had made the same way most of the other recipes online called for, and when it got cold, my butters (and even my salves and lip balms that contained Shea butter) started to get a weird gritty feeling. Now this is not because the product has gone bad, in fact it is still totally usable, it's merely because Shea butter is a gritty butter and will turn this way with rapid temperature changes. If you perform this step when making anything with Shea butter, you will find that it will not turn gritty on you later.

INGREDIENTS

- 1/2 cup unrefined Shea butter (or another kind of butter such as cocoa butter, mango butter, or kokum butter)
- 1/2 cup unrefined mango butter (or another kind of butter such as cocoa butter, kokum butter, or more Shea butter)
- 1/2 cup unrefined coconut oil
- 1/2 cup liquid oil or any combination of liquid carrier oils (such as almond, hemp seed, rosehip seed, sunflower seed, grapeseed, olive, etc.)
- 2 Tbsp. arrowroot powder (optional – helps the oils from the body butter to sink into the skin faster, leaving a less greasy feeling)
- 1 tsp. vitamin e (optional – helps to moisturize skin and to keep the oils from going rancid longer)

DIRECTIONS

- Combine the butters and coconut oil in a double boiler (or makeshift one with a Pyrex/glass bowl over a pan of water) and melt.
- Once mixture has completely melted, start a timer for 20 minutes and let the butters stay at the melted temperature until the timer beeps.
- After 20 minutes, remove from heat and pour into a bowl to cool quickly in an ice bath. (larger bowl underneath filled with ice and water to help the bowl above it, cool quicker.)
- In a separate smaller container, combine liquid oils, vitamin e, and arrowroot powder. It's easiest to combine the arrowroot powder into the oil with a fork.
- When it looks like the butter is half way hardened, meaning there is still a small pool of liquid on top, pour in the liquid oil/arrowroot powder concoction and take out your electric hand mixer or emulsion blender.
- Blend until there are no chunks of hardened butter left. This can not be done by hand. I usually take a spoon and chip away the bottom pieces first to make it easier to blend in the final result.
- If you added the liquid oils too soon and it's still not solid enough to pour into your containers, put the bowl of body butter mixture back onto the ice bath for a minute or two more then blend with it there in the ice bath.
- Spoon butter into the containers that you plan to store the butter in.
- If adding essential oils, this would be the point that you would add them into the butter. I like to add them into each container individually so that I can tailor make the butter's scent to the person I am giving it to!
- The consistency of the butter will be more solidified into it's true consistency, over night.

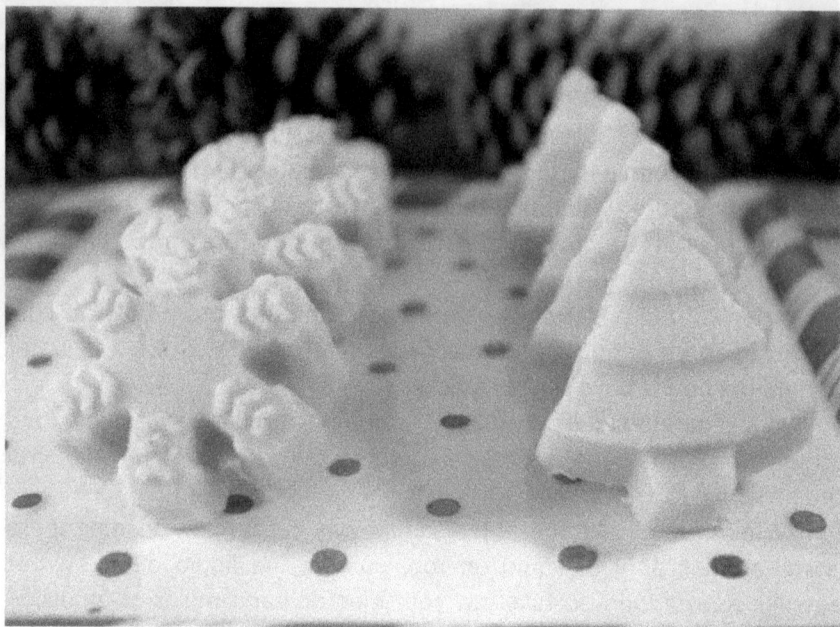

Hard Body Butter Bars

These body butter bars are extremely cute and can be made to fit any of your gifting needs. You can change up the silicon molds depending on what theme you are trying to achieve and even scent the body butter bars according to the likes of your friends and family members. I scented these with peppermint and vanilla, and let me tell you, the Hippy Hubby almost ate them up because they "smelled like peppermint bark". For the gentlemen in your life, you can also scent these with something like peppermint pine, or even leave them unscented. Shea butter has a nice light nutty scent that guys tend to love.

These bars are easy to use and extremely moisturizing to the skin. They will moisturize even the driest of skin on elbows and knees, and even help with heels and feet. The butters and oils will start to warm up and melt when you hold this bar in your hands, then you can rub it all over your body.

INGREDIENTS

- 1/2 cup butter (I like to mix it up and do a combination of butters such as Shea, mango, and cocoa butters)

- 1/2 cup coconut oil (you can substitute some of this for a liquid oil if you so choose BUT if you do that you need to add more beeswax to keep the bar's hardness. I did 1/4 cup coconut oil, 1/4 cup hemp seed oil, and an EXTRA 1/4 cup of beeswax)
- 1/2 cup beeswax (If you want a softer body butter bar, use less beeswax. If you want a harder body butter bar then use more beeswax)
- essential oils for scent (This is optional but definitely makes even better! I used a combination of 20 peppermint essential oil and 15 drops vanilla absolute and it came out smelling like peppermint bark! I had to keep my hubby from eating them!)

DIRECTIONS

• Add all of your butters, coconut oil, and beeswax into your double boiler and melt down. Once melted, allow to sit there on the heat for 20 minutes (as I told you in my diy whipped body butter post, this processes the butters so that they don't get gritty when the temperature changes).

• Remove from heat. If adding essential oils, stir them in.

• Pour into molds. For quick cooling you can put them into the freezer, otherwise these should sit and harden for 4-6 hours.

• If you did not like the consistency and want to add more beeswax, you can pop all of these into your double boiler and melt them down, then add more beeswax and repeat step 3.

• Wrap in wax paper or compostable cellophane and tie with pretty ribbons or twine. Gift to anyone and everyone who has dry skin! (that's pretty much everyone who has skin!)

Body Lotion

Lotion can sometimes be a tricky concoction to make, because unlike body butter, it is an emulsification of oil and water. Combining the two can be a difficult task, considering oil and water do not mix. There is leeway to vary in your recipe as to your ingredients, the most important part is to follow the instructions carefully, otherwise your lotion may not emulsify properly, and will separate. It's OK! It just takes practice! This recipe can be made with just the first 5 ingredients, the last 3 ingredients are to help preserve the lotion, to give it a longer shelf life. With preservation, this lotion will last 4-6 weeks outside of the fridge. If stored in the fridge, this lotion will last up to 3 months!

INGREDEINTS

- ¾ cup carrier oil (Almond, olive, coconut, hemp seed, etc. Be aware that using coconut oil, the lotion will harden when kept in the fridge.)
- 1 Tbsp. Butter (I like to use Shea butter, mango butter, or cocoa butter)
- 3 Tbsp. Beeswax
- 1 cup distilled water (You can use hydrosol, witch hazel, coconut milk, aloe Vera juice, or herbal tea in place of the water)
- 1 tsp. Honey
- 1/8 tsp. Citric acid
- ½ tsp colloidal silver
- ½ tsp. Vitamin e

DIRECTIONS

•   Combine carrier oil, butter, and beeswax in a double boiler. Heat until melted and leave on heat for 20 minutes to process the butter. After 20 minutes, remove from the heat.

•   While the oil mixture is sitting on the heat, bring your distilled water (or other chosen liquid mixture) to a boil and remove from the heat. Stir in citric acid.

•   Allow both the oil mixture and the water to cool to 120 degrees. They should be around the same temperature for the next steps.

•   Mix the vitamin e into the oil mixture.

•   Stir in the honey and colloidal silver into the water mixture.

•   Pour your water mixture into a food processor or blender and turn it on. This can be done in a bowl with a hand mixer, if you don't have a food processor or blender in your home.

•   With your food processor running, VERY slowly pour your oil mixture into the blender. This step is very critical to the mixture emulsifying and not separating. If the oil and water are mixed too quickly, they will separate.

•   Once combined, let the lotion rest for an hour to completely cool, stirring every 15 minutes or so to release any trapped air bubbles.

•   Once completely cooled, store in a lotion pump container or jars in a cool dark place. This lotion will keep even longer, if kept in the fridge.

Moisturizing Body Wash

Though a good bar soap is easy to use in the shower, it is a much more involved process to create on your own than making your own body wash. With the help of liquid castile soap, you can make a great moisturizing body wash that's works very well on a loofa or poof. You can switch up the essential oils (or use none at all), but be sure to use them with care and safely!

- **INGREDEINTS**

- 2/3 cup liquid castile soap
- ¼ cup raw unfiltered honey
- ¼ cup aloe Vera gel
- 1 Tbsp. Coconut oil (you can substitute another carrier oil here such as hemp seed, almond, olive, etc.)
- 1 tsp. Vitamin e
- 15 drops lavender essential oil
- 15 drops grapefruit essential oil

DIRECTIONS

· Combine ingredients in a squeeze top container and shake well before each use.

TO USE: Squeeze a small dime size amount onto your wash cloth/loofa/poof, wet, and wash!

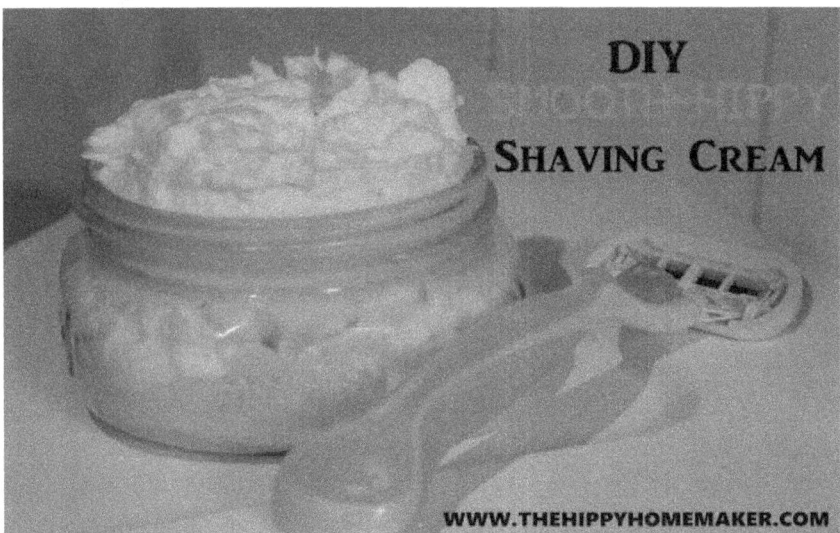

DIY

SHAVING CREAM

WWW.THEHIPPYHOMEMAKER.COM

Shaving Cream

With summertime in full swing, the one thing I can count on is the need to shave my hairy Greek legs to feel that silky smooth feeling that you get when you stick your freshly shaven legs between fresh cool bed sheets on a warm summer night. I truly love that feeling, but it's hard to shave without a good shaving cream to help protect your skin from nicks, cuts, and even skin dryness.

What's even worse is that most of the popular brands of shaving creams that are sold in YOUR local grocery stores, are filled with toxic ingredients that are even banned in many other countries. We have talked about this before; your skin is your largest organ and up to 70% of what you put ON your skin can be absorbed into your blood stream.

Smooth Hippy Shaving Cream

This recipe can be used for women and men alike. It's great for shaving legs, faces, bikini lines, arm pits, and more!

INGREDEINTS

- 1 1/2 cups boiling water
- 1/4 cup aloe Vera gel
- 1 bar of castile soap, grated (I like to use Dr. Bronner's bars soaps)
- 2 Tbsp. unrefined coconut oil
- 2 Tbsp. extra virgin olive oil (I love to use a calendula infused oil here to help with healing my skin further!)
- 2 Tbsp. unrefined Shea butter
- squirt of vitamin e (*optional* - this not only helps to further moisturize your skin
- squirt of colloidal silver (*optional* - I like to add this for both it's amazing topical healing abilities as well as to help naturally preserve the finished product)
- 15 drops essential oil (it's important to research the essential oils for this recipe as some can cause irritation to skin and would not be best to use while shaving)

DIRECTIONS

•   In a double boiler, melt your coconut oil, Shea butter, and olive oil together. Let sit on the heat for 20 minutes once melted, to help prevent the Shea butter from turning gritty later.

- While your butter/oils are heating up in the double boiler, bring your water to a boil. Remove water from heat and add aloe Vera gel and grated bar soap in a large bowl. Stir until soap is completely dissolved. Let soapy water mixture sit on the counter to cool.
- Once your 20 minutes is up on the butter/oils, remove from heat and allow to cool.
- Once both oil mixture and water mixture are both cooled a bit (around 100 degrees or warm enough for the butters to still be melted), we are going to mix them together the same way we would if we were making a lotion. That is to say, get out your food processor/blender/hand mixer. I am using my hand mixer for this but you can do this in your large food processor or blender if that is what you have on hand. No matter the method, you're going to blend while pouring the butter/oil mixture slowly into the soapy water mixture. Once combined, you can blend in the vitamin e and colloidal silver if you are using either.
- If you were impatient and happened to blend them into one another too soon (meaning they are still too liquidy and haven't cooled enough to be a thick whipped cream like texture), don't fret. I get impatient all the time and this is how I deal with it. Make an ice bath in a separate larger bowl and put your shaving cream mixture's bowl in the ice bath. Every 3-5 minutes or so blend it with your hand blender until you get the thickness and consistency you were looking for.
- Whether you were impatient or not, this shaving cream will be completely finished processing itself over night. You can use it as soon as you are finished making it, but it will get a little bit thicker and foamier as it cool completely overnight.
- Store in a glass mason jar. This recipe fills (2) 1-Quart mason jars.

TO USE: Scoop out a hand full of shaving cream, lather up wet legs, shave, and rinse! If you're shaving your face, you can always follow with a really great homemade aftershave! If you are shaving your legs or bikini area then follow up with my REALLY AMAZING homemade body butter! I have found that consistently using my body butter on my legs right after shaving in the shower, has helped my hair to grow back thinner, softer, and less often.

Body Scrubs

The key to softy silky smooth skin, is exfoliation. I can remember the very first time that I used a sugar scrub. My hands had never felt that soft. I was in complete awe! The best part is they are extremely easy to make at home! You can make any of these scrubs with sea salt instead of sugar, but I prefer sugar. Sugar scrubs are one of the best ways to revitalize your skin all over your body. Sugar is a natural humectant, helping to hydrate your skin and to hold moisture in. Sugar is also a natural source of glycolic acid, an alpha hydroxy acid that penetrates the skin and breaks down the "glue" that bonds skin cells, encouraging cell turnover and generating fresher, younger-looking skin. Glycolic acid is typically used to treat sun-damaged and aging skin as well.

There are many variations that you can do with these scrubs. You can add different finely ground freeze dried fruits, use honey instead of oil, or add different herbs and essential oils to customize this to your own preferences.

Base Sugar Scrub

INGREDEINTS

- 1 cup sugar
- ¼ cup carrier oil (olive oil, almond oil, coconut oil, hemp seed oil, honey etc.)
- 1 tsp. Vitamin e
- 10-20 drops essential oil (be sure to research all essential oils you choose to use to avoid irritation of the skin.)

DIRECTIONS

• Combine ingredients in a bowl and keep in a sealed jar. Store in a cool dark place. To keep this sugar scrub longer, avoid introducing water into the scrub. Always use clean dry hands or a spoon, and keep sealed when not in use.

TO USE: Using dry hands, scoop out a small amount of scrub and rub all over body to exfoliate and moisturize your skin.

Grapefruit Coffee Cellulite Scrub

This scrub is very popular with my clients! It's one of my best-selling sugar scrubs. The caffeine in the coffee grounds helps improve circulation, which will remove excess water from skin and make it appear firmer. When caffeine is absorbed into the skin, it acts as a tightening agent. This helps reduce cellulite over time. Rubbing grounds into your skin will slough off dead skin cells and leave your skin feeling refreshed. It also helps reduce puffiness and swelling, to make your skin glow. Grapefruit essential oil not only awakens the senses and brightens the mood but it also is used to help combat fat and cellulite.

INGREDEINTS

- 1 cup sugar
- ¼ cup ground coffee
- 2 Tbsp. Almond oil
- 2 Tbsp. Avocado oil
- 25 drops grapefruit essential oil
- 1 tsp. Vitamin e

DIRECTIONS

•   Combine ingredients in a bowl, stirring until everything is properly blended together. Store in a jar.

TO USE: Scrub over thighs, butt, and anywhere else where cellulite might be a problem!

Flower Power Sugar Scrub

I love this florally herbal sugar scrub! I find the sweet floral scent to be delightful to my senses, while in the shower! It brings memories of spring time meadows to mind.

INGREDEINTS

- 1 cup sugar
- 2 Tbsp. Almond oil
- 2 Tbsp. Rosehip seed oil
- 2 Tbsp. Lavender buds
- 2 Tbsp. Ground chamomile flowers
- 2 Tbsp. Lightly ground rose petals
- 5 drops roman chamomile essential oil
- 5 drops rose absolute
- 20 drops lavender essential oil
- 2 drops ylang ylang essential oil

DIRECTIONS

•   Combine ingredients in a bowl, stirring until everything is properly blended together. Store in a jar.

TO USE: Using dry hands, scoop out a small amount of scrub and rub all over body to exfoliate and moisturize your skin.

Good Morning Sunshine Sugar Scrub

I just love the smell of citrus in the morning! All citrus scents are so uplifting and happy, that starting my day with a zesty citrus sugar scrub is so invigorating and wakes me up! I love to use fresh citrus zest for this recipe, though you can use ground dried citrus peel in its place. You can also switch up any of the citrus for other citrus of your choosing!

INGREDIENTS

- 1 cup sugar
- 2 Tbsp. Rosehip seed oil
- 2 Tbsp. Hemp seed oil
- 1 Tbsp. Lemon zest
- 1 Tbsp. Orange zest
- 1 Tbsp. Lime zest

Soothing Bath Salts

After a stressful day at work or with the kiddos, all that you want to do is relax in a hot bath and let your cares melt away. Baths have been long since used for more than just luxurious getaways. They are used to help ailing muscles, heal the sick, detoxify the body, cure skin conditions, and so much more!

Our skins, the largest organ in/on our body, absorb up to 75% of what we put onto it. That means that we can utilize the healing benefits of specific herbs, flowers, and barks to give us the natural healing benefits that those specific herbs impart. For maximum healing benefit to the mind, body, and soul, you can combine salts, herbs, and moisturizing oils in your bath.

EPSOM SALTS – The healing benefits of Epsom salt baths dates back to 1618, when a farmer in Epsom England discovered his cows were unhappy drinking the water due to its bitter taste. He noticed that the water healed scratches and rashes and it didn't take long before word of mouth spread the word. Epsom salts are made mostly of magnesium and sulphates.

Taking an Epsom bath can help with the following:

- ease stress and improve sleep
- support muscle and nerve functions

- help prevent artery hardening and blood clots
- reduce inflammation to relieve pain and muscle cramps
- improve oxygen use and energy levels
- flush toxins and contaminants from the body
- improve absorption of nutrients
- help prevent or ease migraine headaches
- softens and exfoliates the skin

BATH TEAS – Salts aren't the only way to help heal the body, improve the skin, and relax the mind. Herbs have been long known to have many different healing benefits. Not only is lavender known to calm and sooth the mind, it's also highly antibacterial, antiviral, and even anti-inflammatory. Such tidbits of knowledge can help you to find many different healing benefits just from the teas that you have in your kitchen pantry. Green tea has been know to have many healing benefits to the skin, body, and even metabolism. Chamomile of course, is known for it's comforting and calming effects; but is also a great anti-inflammatory, as well as gas and upset tummy reliever. Peppermint can help cool a sunburn, and eucalyptus can help ease chest congestion.

You can either add herbs straight to your bath, or for an easier cleanup fill large cloth tea bags with your herbal mixture and drop it into the tub.

Soothing Bath Salts Base Recipe

INGREDEINTS

- 1-2 cups Epsom salt (you can combine other sea salts with this including dead sea, pink Himalayan, etc.)
- ¼ cup herbs of choice (lavender, chamomile, dandelion, rose, rosemary, etc.)
- 10-15 drops essential oil (*optional* – please know the essential oils that you are using in your bath salts as some essential oils are potential irritants and should not be used in the bath. Some great essential oils for baths are lavender, chamomile, tangerine, sweet orange, lemon, sweet marjoram, ylang ylang, rose, jasmine, cypress, juniper berry)

DIRECTIONS

- Combine ingredients in a bowl. Sprinkle into your bath or bath tea bag; soak & enjoy!

Hair of the Dog Bath Salts

These bath salts were originally created for my husband. He is a big fan of drinking craft beers and sometimes that means he is feeling it the next morning. Sometimes that leads to a morning full of headaches, loud noises, and nauseated stomachs. One morning I decided to make him a bath salt combination that would help ease the tension and nausea as well as get much needed vitamins and minerals back into his body.

These bath salts contain a special blend of herbs that are detoxifying to the liver and very high in the electrolytes that your body needs to get over a hangover faster. This is also a favorite among my clientele.

INGREDEINTS

- ½ cup Epsom salt
- ½ cup dead sea salt
- 2 Tbsp. Rose hips
- 2 Tbsp. Oatstraw
- 2 Tbsp. Nettle
- 2 Tbsp. Dandelion
- 5 drops ginger essential oil
- 15 drops sweet orange essential oil
- 10 drops lavender essential oil
- 10 drops lemon essential oil

DIRECTIONS

•   Combine ingredients in a bowl. Sprinkle into your bath or bath tea bag; soak & enjoy!

Hippy Cleanse Herbal Bath Salts

These bath salts were made for detoxing. If you are going on a cleanse or detoxifying your body, these are a great addition to help cleanse your body of toxins!

INGREDIENTS

- ½ cup Epsom salt
- ½ cup dead sea salt (you can substitute this with more Epsom salt if you do not have this on hand.)
- 2 Tbsp. Bentonite clay

- 2 Tbsp. Green tea
- 10 drops lemon essential oil
- 15 drops grapefruit essential oil
- 5 drops juniper berry essential oil
- 10 drops lavender essential oil

DIRECTIONS

- Combine ingredients in a bowl. Sprinkle into your bath or bath tea bag; soak & enjoy!

Muscle Soothing Herbal Bath Salts

After a hard work out or a tough move, some muscle relief is always welcome. These bath salts were designed specifically with muscle pains, strains, and pulls in mind. Submerse your aching body in minerals, herbs, and essential oils combined to relieve your body's aches and pains.

INGREDIENTS

- 1 cup Epsom salt
- 1 Tbsp. Rosemary
- 1 Tbsp. Lemonbalm
- 1 Tbsp. St. John's Wort
- 1 Tbsp. Comfrey
- 5 drops rosemary essential oil
- 15 drops lavender essential oil
- 5 drops eucalyptus essential oil
- 5 drops roman chamomile essential oil

DIRECTIONS

- Combine ingredients in a bowl. Sprinkle into your bath or bath tea bag; soak & enjoy!

Good Night Sleep Tight Herbal Bath Salts

Sleep is such a treasured thing, and sometimes it's hard to come by. Good Night Sleep Tight was created to help aid in calming the mind and body, to effectively help you sleep better without the worry of a groggy morning.

I designed these bath salts to be an easy, effective, and natural method of relieving insomnia and aiding in falling asleep faster, and sleeping deeper. Good Night Sleep Tight's calming blend of lavender, chamomile, Valerian root, hops, passionflower and essential oils of lavender, chamomile, ylang ylang, and sweet marjoram will help shut off the busy brain and allow your body to relax into a much needed slumber.

INGREDEINTS

- 1 cup Epsom salts
- 2 Tbsp. Lavender buds
- 2 Tbsp. Chamomile
- 1 Tbsp. Valerian root
- 1 Tbsp. Passion flower
- 1 Tbsp. Hops
- 15 drops lavender essential oil
- 10 drops roman chamomile essential oil
- 2 drops ylang ylang essential oil
- 5 drops sweet marjoram essential oil
- 5 drops bergamot essential oil
- 2 drops Valerian essential oil

DIRECTIONS

- Combine ingredients in a bowl. Sprinkle into your bath or bath tea bag; soak & enjoy!

Take a Chill Pill Herbal Bath Salts

After a long hard day at work (or at home taking care of the kiddos!), all that you want is some stress-relieving "ME time". Take-a-Chill-Pill Calming Bath Salts was specially formulated with ultimate relaxation in mind.

Take a Chill Pill is a Hippy Homemaker blend that I came up with to help calm my son in the evenings. It is a calming blend of lavender, chamomile, tangerine, and vanilla. It helps to relax, soothe, and calm anyone down during any time of the day.

INGREDIENTS

- 1 cup Epsom salts
- 2 Tbsp. Lavender buds

- 2 Tbsp. Chamomile
- 15 drops lavender essential oil
- 6 drops roman chamomile essential oil
- 10 drops tangerine essential oil
- 4 drops vanilla absolute

DIRECTIONS

• Combine ingredients in a bowl. Sprinkle into your bath or bath tea bag; soak & enjoy!

Oatmeal Bath

I originally created this oatmeal bath as a replacement for the Aveeno oatmeal bath packets. I usually put a bottle of this in the baby gift baskets that I give at baby showers. This oatmeal bath is great for sensitive baby skin, rashes, poison oak and ivy, eczema, and more!

INGREDEINTS

• ¾ cup finely ground oats (It's easiest to use a food processor for this)
• ½ cup baking soda
• ¼ cup coconut milk powder (*optional* – this helps to moisturize and heal the skin)
• 20 drops lavender essential oil
• 10 drops roman chamomile essential oil

DIRECTIONS

• Combine ingredients and store in an air tight jar. Sprinkle desired amount into bath and soak for at least 15 minutes to help relieve itching, burning, and soften skin.

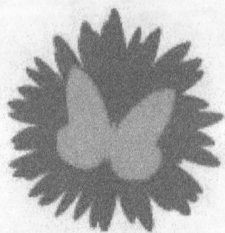

Chapter Five

Toiletries & My Natural Medicine Cabinet

It's extremely empowering to me, to be able to make my family's toiletries and natural healing salves. I have at this point completely cut out my spending at the grocery store for toiletries. I really enjoy being able to make whatever we might need, on the fly. You can literally make everything from deodorant and toothpaste to owie cream and vapor rubs. Everything you need can easily be made at home for a fraction of the price.

The recipes for the herbal infused oils that I use in many of these healing salves, can be found in chapter 10.

Toothpaste

Most toothpastes on the market, including many of the natural ones, are filled with sulfates, parabens, and even fluoride (which has been found to not help the teeth in any manner, as previously thought, and is highly toxic!!!).

This toothpaste is safe to use with toddlers as well, though I would half the amount of essential oils and only stick to tangerine or sweet orange to flavor the toothpaste for a child under the age of 6. Make without essential oils for children under the age of two. If your child has not learned to spit out the toothpaste, do not use essential oils. If you are making this for your dog, use only half the peppermint called for or none at all. For pets toothpaste, DO NOT sweeten with Xylitol. It is toxic to dogs and cats.

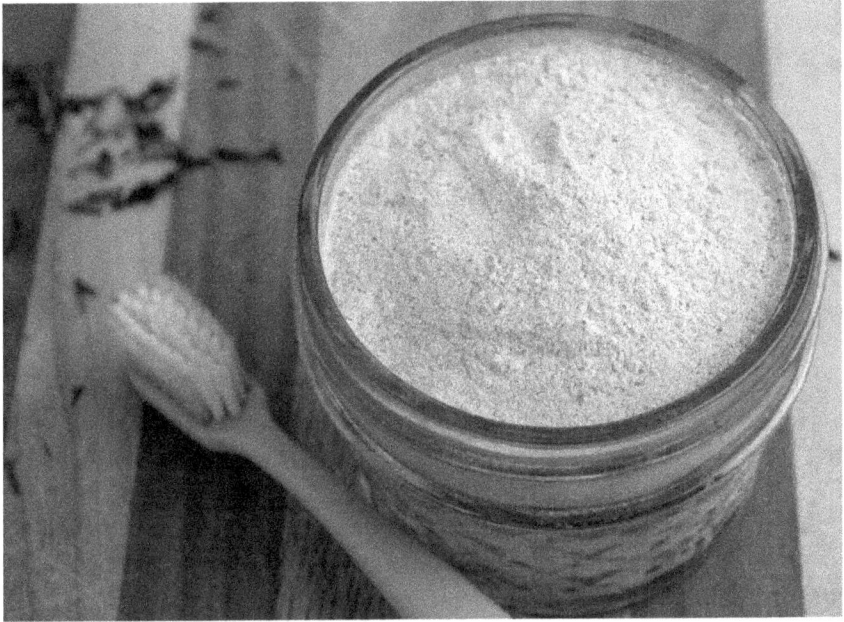

Flavor Options

Peppermint (the classic)

Cinnamint (half peppermint essential oil, half cinnamon leaf essential oil)

Spearmint

Sweet Orange (Tasty kid's toothpaste)

Tangerine (My favorite tasty kid's toothpaste)

Grapefruit

Lemon (This would also give a slight whitening power to the toothpaste)

Fresh Mint (half/half of spearmint and peppermint)

Peppermint Lavender (tasty AND antibacterial/anti-viral)

Grapefruit Lavender (It wouldn't be Hippy Homemaker without this flavor...)

INGREDEINTS

- 1/2 cup coconut oil
- 1/4 cup baking soda (you can add more to this recipe, some recipes call for equal parts coconut oil and baking soda, but I

feel that it's too abrasive and salty tasting. It is up to you, you can change it's consistency to you and your family's liking!)
- 30-60 drops essential oils
- 2-4 Tbsp. Xylitol (sweeten to taste, this stuff is good for your teeth so you can not go wrong with it! Note: If you are making this for your pets, don't sweeten at all. Xylitol is TOXIC to dogs and cats!)

DIRECTIONS

• Combine coconut oil and baking soda (keep in mind this will be a softer paste in the summer and a harder paste in the winter, if you melt the coconut oil before you make this, keep in mind you will have to blend/stir the entire thing completely once it has cooled completely and come to room temperature.) until blended together.

• Add essential oil and Xylitol to taste. Keep in a mason jar with a lid, and dip toothbrush into toothpaste BEFORE wetting with water. (If water gets into the toothpaste it may inevitably bring bacteria with it!)

Remineralizing Herbal Toothpowder

When I made my first batch of tooth powder, I was looking to try something new and herbal for my oral hygiene. After reading through one of my Rosemary Gladstar books, I decided I wanted to try out a tooth powder. The idea sounded fairly easy to make and use.

I must admit, going from a toothpaste to a tooth powder, I was a little apprehensive about brushing my teeth...with mud. The first time that I used my tooth powder, I was most definitely weirded out. It even LOOKS like you are brushing your teeth with mud...but please don't let that detour you! Seriously, once you get passed the fact that you no longer need foaming soapy bubbles in your mouth, and realize how fresh and clean your mouth is, you will be hooked on tooth powder!

Ingredients for a healthier mouth

Most people are quite aware of the use of baking soda in oral health care, but there are many other natural and effective herbal remedies to use along side baking soda, for a fresher and cleaner mouth.

• Bentonite clay - Rich in bone feeding minerals such as calcium and potassium, bentonite clay is a fabulous non-toxic teeth cleaner! Not only can you take bentonite clay internally for detoxifying purposes, but the high mineral content that this clay contains also helps to re-mineralize the teeth! NOTE: Do not house this in anything metal (including the lid) or use metal utensils when using bentonite clay. Bentonite clay is negatively charged (the reason it's able to absorb and purify toxins in the body) and when it touches metal, the positive charge deactivates some of it's amazing benefits.

• Myrrh gum powder - This highly antibacterial, anti-fungal, and antiseptic gum resin has been used for centuries to heal many different diseases, but one thing that it is well known to help with is dental care! Using Myrrh in your tooth care routine can help to prevent gingivitis, heal all sorts of gum problems, and is known to be an immune booster.

• Mint - The use of mint in oral hygiene is actually rather new. Over time, many cultures used what was around them in their natural habitats for breath fresheners and tooth scrubs (i.e. parsley, rosemary, sage, fennel seeds, cardamom, star anise, clove, etc.) but the idea to mostly use mint came about with the introduction of toothpaste in the late 1800's. Peppermint is a known digestive aid, making a cup of peppermint tea do double duty when you drink it after dinner!

• Cloves - Highly anti-fungal and antibacterial, this fragrant and spicy herb is well known in the dental world. It's known to help relieve tooth and gum pain and is even used toothache oils used by natural dentists.

• Baking soda - A wonderful abrasive to help clean teeth, baking soda has many benefits to using it in oral health care. Baking soda not only helps to clean teeth but can be used, dissolved in water, as a mouthwash as well.

• Xylitol - According to xylitol.org "research done in widely different conditions confirms that xylitol use significantly reduces tooth decay rates both in high-risk groups (high caries prevalence, poor nutrition, and poor oral hygiene) and in low-risk groups (low caries incidence using all current prevention recommendations)." Note – Keep out of reach of DOGS and CATS. Xylitol is TOXIC to DOGS and CATS.

Why a tooth powder over a toothpaste?

Tooth powders have actually been around a lot longer than tooth paste. Many ancient peoples used to cleanse their teeth by chewing on chalk and clays. This eventually evolved into a tooth powder, and now today with all of our herbal knowledge, they are easily adapted for oral health and hygiene.

The great thing about a tooth powder is that it does not change it's state depending on the weather, it's very easy to take with you in a small jar no matter where you might be traveling to, and it keeps for longer than any paste because it's made with dry ingredients. You can even combine this recipe with coconut oil for a remineralizing toothpaste if you just can't handle the powder.

Alternate flavor choices

You don't have to use peppermint flavor for your tooth powder flavoring! You can use a whole host of flavors, just replace the herb and essential oils in the recipe with these options:

- Spearmint - spearmint leaf and spearmint essential oil
- Minty Fresh - (1/2 each) spearmint leaf and peppermint leaf, essential oils of spearmint and peppermint
- Peppermint Sage - (1/2 each) peppermint leaf and sage leaf, essential oils of peppermint and sage
- Cinnamon & Cloves - clove powder, cinnamon leaf and clove essential oil
- Cinnamint Spice - (1/2 of each) clove powder and peppermint leaf powder, essential oils of cinnamon leaf, clove, and peppermint
- Oranges & Clove - clove powder, essential oils of clove and sweet orange
- Citrus Mint - spearmint leaf powder, essential oils of sweet orange, grapefruit, and spearmint
- Vanilla Mint - peppermint leaf powder, essential oil of peppermint, and vanilla extract
- Rosemary Lime - rosemary powder, essential oils of lime peel and rosemary
- Citrus - Any single or combination of citrus peel powder, essential oils of (single or combined) lemon, sweet orange, grapefruit, and/or lime

INGREDEINTS

- 1 cup bentonite clay
- 1/4 cup baking soda
- 2 Tbsp. myrrh gum powder
- 2 Tbsp. finely ground peppermint leaf powder (or other herb choice)
- 2 Tbsp. ground stevia leaf (optional, I am talking about the real plant, not the sugar replacement from the grocery store. You can substitute this for more xylitol powder)

- 2 Tbsp. finely ground xylitol powder (optional, you can substitute this for more stevia leaf powder if you don't have)
- 5-10 drops peppermint essential oil

DIRECTIONS

- Grind your herbs and xylitol into a smooth powder. Combine all of the powdered ingredients and then mix in essential oils. I personally find it easiest to mix the essential oils in with my fingers. Store in a mason jar with a plastic lid. (I use these in my home)
- To use, apply a small amount of tooth powder to your tooth brush, wet gently with a few drops of water and brush teeth normally as you would with toothpaste. Rinse well. (I usually get a couple drops of water on my toothbrush just to get it wet, then dip it gently into the powder and then get a couple more drops of water onto my brush to wet the powder completely. Then I brush away!)
- Follow with your homemade mouthwash!

Mouthwash

In our household, we used to use Listerine to rinse our mouths out. It was always a harsh and painful experience to rinse my mouth out with mouthwash. When I decided to start making my own mouthwash, I was intent upon making a mouthwash that wasn't so harsh on my mouth. To do that, I needed to avoid alcohol and use peroxide.

Hydrogen peroxide – the key to a fresh white smile

Hydrogen Peroxide is a known disinfectant and bleach, and is used in all sorts of ways to clean throughout my house naturally. Not only is hydrogen peroxide a proven weapon in the fight against most bacteria as well as a gentle whitener for teeth, it's also been shown to fight gingivitis. One study published by the National Institutes of Health found that when used as a mouth rinse, Hydrogen peroxide prevents bacteria buildup and plaque, both contributors to gingivitis. The other awesome thing about using hydrogen peroxide in your mouthwash, is that it does an amazing job at helping to heal canker sores too! Take that alcohol! (Honestly though, I used to get canker sores all the time before I changed my diet and lifestyle, and I now I can't actually remember having a single canker sore since we went hippy. It is important to remember that your mouthwash may help heal the canker sores up, but the underlying cause, may in fact be your diet.)

Most conventional mouthwashes contain toxic

ingredients

The most popular brands of mouthwash may not even be the best dental options. Many contain ingredients that are known to be toxic and unhealthy such sodium lauryl sulfate, pthalates, and parabens. Mouthwashes are also most often sweetened with artificial sugars such as sodium saccharin (a known carcinogen) and sucralose, which has been known to trigger migraines and other issues. These mouthwashes also contain synthetic flavors and colors such as FD&C Blue 1 and FD&C Green 3.

Why not alcohol-based mouthwash?

Most mouthwashes on the market, natural included, are often alcohol-based, containing anywhere from 18 to 26% alcohol. Mouthwashes containing alcohol that are used regularly, can contribute to cancers of the mouth, tongue, and throat. In 2009, a review in the Dental Journal of Australia confirmed that alcohol-based mouthwashes contribute to an increased risk of oral cancers.

Use of mouthwashes containing alcohol will temporarily reduce bad breath, but in the long term they help to improve conditions for the development of bad breath because they dry the mouth out. The continued production of saliva is key to keeping the mouth fresh.

INGREDEINTS

- 1 cup distilled water/peppermint hydrosol (You can use just plain distilled water here, but I love to use peppermint hydrosol instead of water because it adds a great deal of extra yummy flavor, smell, and healing properties from the peppermint herbs hydrosol is distilled from)
- 1 cup 3% hydrogen peroxide (It MUST be 3% and no more, otherwise it could be hazardous to your health, 3% is found in most grocery stores and is the most common peroxide sold on the shelves.)
- 1 Tbsp. Xylitol (a natural sweetener that is known to help prevent cavities and gum disease)
- 5-10 drops peppermint essential oil (depending on personal strength and taste. We actually use 5 drops peppermint and 5 drops spearmint in ours)

DIRECTIONS

• Combine ingredients in a dark glass bottle or re-use a hydrogen peroxide bottle, and shake to dissolve the xylitol. Peroxide breaks down in sunlight, so storing in a dark container in a cool dark place is imperative to keeping your peroxide from turning into water.

• Shake before use, then swish around and gargle in your freshly brushed mouth for 2 minutes. Spit and rinse with water. DO NOT SWALLOW MOUTHWASH, SPIT OUT AFTER USE.

NOTES: You can switch out the essential oils (and hydrosol if using) for other essential oils including peppermint clove, spearmint, sweet orange, grapefruit, tangerine, lemon, sage, rosemary, and cilantro.

• You can effectively gargle with peppermint tea for a cleaner mouth and fresher breath.

• a tsp. of baking soda in 8 oz. water with a few drops of essential oil can also be used as a natural mouthwash.

• a Tbsp. of apple cider vinegar in 8 oz. water with a few drops of essential oil has also known to be a great mouthwash (if you can handle the vinegar flavor)

Strawberry Honey Tooth Brightener

This is the most delicious way to brush your teeth! Strawberries contain a mild bleaching agent that, if used often, will whiten and brighten your teeth! This is a much safer option to use than lemon juice because lemon juice is too acidic for your tooth enamel. Honey naturally has a small amount of peroxide in it and is a known antibacterial and antiseptic, making it perfect to brush your teeth with!

INGREIENTS

• 1 medium sized ripe strawberry
• ½ Tbsp. Raw unfiltered honey

DIRECTIONS

• In a food processor, puree strawberry and honey together until it's a nice pulp. Dip your toothbrush into the tasty mixture and brush your teeth as normal. Rinse your mouth thoroughly afterward.

Charcoal Tooth Whitener

This is one of the most surprising recipes to me. Not only do you look like your making your mouth much dirtier when you do this, but your teeth actually come out noticeably whiter after using this tooth whitener. I honestly was shocked the first time that I tried this simple remedy. Activated charcoal is extremely absorbent and when used in the mouth, pulls toxins and stains from your teeth naturally.

INGREDIENTS

- activated charcoal
- toothbrush

DIRECTIONS

•   Wet your toothbrush with water and dip it in the activated charcoal. I usually use the capsules and just open one into a jar.

•   Brush your teeth in gentle circles, with the activated charcoal, for two minutes. Spit out and rinse your mouth really well!

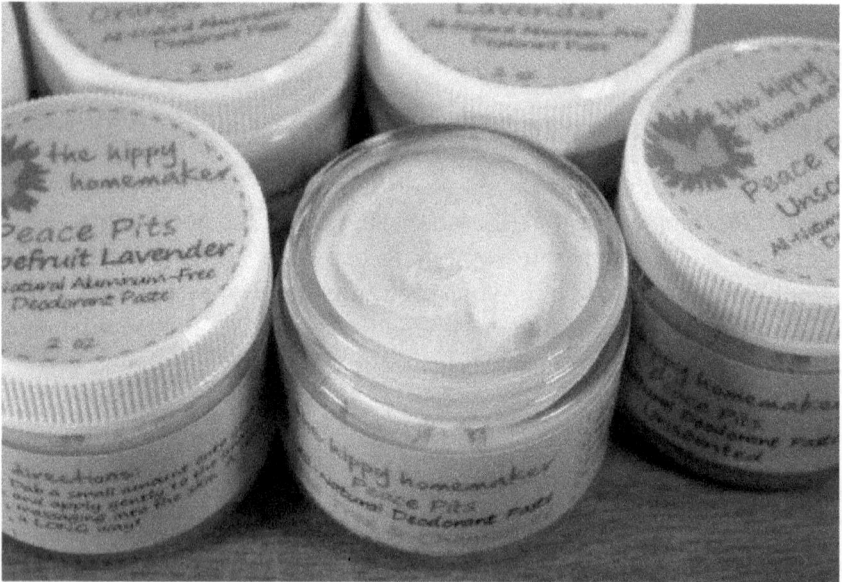

Peace Pits Deodorant Paste

If you told me two years ago that I would be a successful deodorant maker, I would have laughed in your face. When I first made this deodorant I was at my wits end. I had tried all sorts of natural deodorants from the store, and none of them worked all that well. Some had me stinking an hour into using them, while others made my pits feel like they were foaming up. I had stumbled across recipes on the internet that contained coconut oil, baking soda, and arrowroot powder (or cornstarch). I couldn't resist but to try some of these super simple recipes out. After testing them out, I put together my own recipe and perfected it.

All of the natural homemade deodorant recipes out there, describe the process the same; melt and pour. I somehow was gifted with the idea that I could whip my deodorant in the same way I do with body butters. This truly revolutionized the texture of this paste and has made it the BY FAR the best seller in my shoppe. Pretty much every single order has at least one Peace Pits deodorant paste on it, and my clients rave at it's amazing effectiveness!

INGREDEINTS

- ¼ cup unrefined coconut oil
- ¼ cup unrefined Shea butter (*optional* - this helps to soften and heal the skin and makes the baking soda less harsh)
- ¼ cup baking soda
- ¼ cup arrowroot powder (this can be substituted with cornstarch)
- essential oils (*optional* - only a couple drops are needed, though some essential oils should be avoided for use in deodorant as they can cause irritation to the skin.)

DIRECTIONS

•   This recipe works best if you do NOT heat up the coconut oil. If it is rock solid and you can not get away with mixing this up without doing a little bit of heating, do not melt completely, just SOFTEN the oil enough to stir the powders into the coconut oil.

•   In a medium sized mixing bowl, completely stir the baking soda, arrowroot powder, and coconut oil together until the powder has been worked into the oil. It will seem at first that there is too much powder and not enough oil, just keep stirring and it will begin to come together.

•   In a double boiler heat the Shea butter until melted. Allow to sit on heat for 20 minutes to process the Shea butter.

•   Pour the Shea butter into the bowl with the coconut oil/baking soda mixture. Place bowl in an ice bath to cool quickly.

- When it looks like the deodorant is half way hardened, meaning there is still a small pool of liquid on top, pour in the vitamin e and take out your electric hand mixer or emulsion blender.
- I usually use the whisk attachment on my electric hand mixer, blend until there are no chunks of hardened deodorant left. This can not be done by hand. I usually take a spoon and chip away the bottom pieces first to make it easier to blend in the final result.
- If you blended too soon and it's still not solid enough to pour into a container, put the bowl of deodorant back onto the ice bath for a minute or two more then blend with it there in the ice bath.
- Spoon deodorant into the container that you plan to store it in.
- If adding essential oils, this would be the point that you would add them into the deodorant.
- The consistency of the deodorant will be more solidified into it's true consistency, over night. In the summertime, this deodorant will be soft or liquid. If this is the case, just give it a stir before use. In the wintertime the coconut oil and Shea butter will solidify, which makes it easier to use as a paste.

Calendula Antiseptic Owie Cream

The very first healing salve that I learned how to make was a calendula salve. This salve has replaced our need to purchase any Neosporin in our house. This salve has been miraculous at healing cuts, scrapes, burns, and even pimples. The secret to this salve is the skin healing herbs that are infused into the oil. You can find the recipes for the herbal infused oils in chapter 10.

INGREDEINTS

- ½ cup herbal infused "magic healing oil" (or coconut/olive oil)
- ¼ cup unrefined Shea butter
- ¼ cup beeswax pastilles
- ¼ tsp. Lavender essential oil
- ¼ tsp. Tea tree essential oil
- 30 drops lemon essential oil

DIRECTIONS

- In a double boiler, melt oil, Shea butter, and beeswax. Once melted, allow to sit on the heat for 20 minutes to process the Shea butter.

- Remove from heat. Add essential oils and then pour into jars or tins for use on all of your owies.

TO USE: Dab a small amount onto your fingers and apply generously to your cuts, scrapes, and other boo boos! Use as often as needed. A little bit goes a LONG way!

Fungus Amungus Anti-Fungal Salve

Fungal infections can be the peskiest kind of infection to get rid of because once they find a host, they like to stick around for the long haul. Though you can cure fungal infections using salves, creams, and sprays, diet is also a major factor in helping to clear a fungus from your body. A diet high in sugar and yeast will lead to an overgrowth of yeast within the body, causing a fungal infection. A more alkaline whole foods diet is recommended to help aid in ridding your body completely of the fungus.

Along with a diet change there are a few other things you can do to get rid of that pesky fungus. My favorite natural treatment is an anti-fungal salve. With a salve I can combine the natural healing properties of herbs, essential oils, carrier oils, butters, and more! Salves are also highly moisturizing to the skin so they make skin repair much quicker than it would with a convention pharmaceutical treatment.

Essential oils with anti-fungal properties

There are a ton of essential oils that in combination can battle even the toughest of fungal infections. Some are more irritating than others to the skin so please be sure to research which essential oils you are adding to your salve.

- oregano
- thyme
- clove
- lavender
- tea tree
- geranium
- chamomile
- cedarwood
- cinnamon bark
- Frankincense
- lemongrass
- pine

- ravensara
- rosemary

Healing fungal infections with herbs is simple

There are many herbs that are very helpful to healing a fungal infection, but the two that are most notable and usually can be found in the best of herbal anti-fungal salves are chaparral and black walnut. These two are stand out herbs in the anti-fungal department but there are plenty more herbs that can be used in your salve to help heal fungal infections:

- Chaparral leaf – Not only is chaparral anti-fungal but it is also antibacterial, antiseptic, and anti-parasitic. This herb is jam packed with skin healing properties and packs a powerful punch against fungal infections.
- Black Walnut Hulls - The most commonly used herb in anti-fungal creams and sprays, black walnut hulls are also antibacterial, antiseptic, and anti-parasitic. Any really good herbal salve for fungal infections will have black walnut hulls in it.
- Echinacea - Not only is this herb a super immune booster, which helps aid the body in ridding infections faster, but this super herb is also anti-fungal!
- Cloves - Cloves contain some of the same phenols as Oil of Oregano, which are highly anti-fungal in nature, as well as antimicrobial, antioxidant, antiviral, and anti-inflammatory. This oil has been prized for centuries for its anti-fungal properties.
- Lavender - I really believe that lavender is one of those herbs that is the heal-all end-all "god herbs". This herb is good for so many things, it's not surprising that it is also anti-fungal. What can't lavender do?
- Calendula - One of the best skin healing herbs, calendula is not just great for healing wounds and lacerations but also fungal infections. Calendula is great at reducing inflammation, treating burns, scrapes, eczema, and more!
- Garlic - Not only is garlic one of the most potent natural antibiotics healing anything from ear infections to colds, garlic is also highly anti-fungal. You can throw some garlic into a blender with a little bit of water or oil and rub it onto your feet or infected area. Some people even like to sprinkle garlic powder into their shoes when fighting a foot fungus.

INGREDEINTS

- 1/4 cup beeswax

- 1/4 cup unrefined Shea butter
- 1/2 cup chaparral/black walnut hull infused extra virgin olive oil (For the salve that I sell in my shop, I infuse chaparral, black walnut hulls, echinacea, and calendula into an EV olive oil/EV coconut oil mixture)
- 1/2 tsp. tea tree essential oil
- 1/2 tsp. lavender essential oil
- 20 drops red thyme essential oil
- 20 drops clove essential oil

DIRECTIONS

•   In a double boiler combine beeswax, Shea butter, and herbal infused oil. Melt ingredients.

•   Once ingredients are completely melted, let them sit over the heat for 20 minutes to process the Shea butter.

•   After your 20 minutes are up, remove the double boiler from the heat.

•   Mix in your essential oils and pour into containers to cool. Once cool, store in a dark cool area for maximum shelf life.

TO USE: Apply to a clean and dry affected area two times a day until infection is completely gone. Fungal infections can be very difficult to get rid of, persistence and a healthy diet are the keys.

Other natural treatments to help heal foot fungus

•   Combine one part apple cider vinegar and four parts water, then soak your feet for soothing relief.

•   A combination of sea salts and Epsom salts in a foot soak can be very beneficial to helping heal athlete's foot.

•   A foot powder can be made by combining 4 parts arrowroot powder, 1 part finely ground chaparral leaf, and 1 part finely ground black walnut hulls. Apply to clean dry feet or shoes for all day healing.

•   Always keep affected areas clean and dry, moisture is the leading cause of bacterial and fungal growth.

Cool Vibes Vapor Rub Salve

During the cold and flu season, a good vapor rub can make the difference as to whether or not I get any sleep. Whenever I can't breathe or have a nasty cough, I usually rub this salve all over my feet and then put socks on before going to bed. It may sound kooky, but it works so well that even my doctor suggested doing this to get some better rest at night.

This salve is not for children under the age of 10. The menthol and cineol 1,8 content in the peppermint, eucalyptus, and rosemary are not safe for young children and can cause a slowness of breathing. It is best to use the Cool Vibes Vapor Rub Jr. for children under the age of 10.

INGREDEINTS

- ½ cup olive oil
- ¼ cup unrefined coconut oil (this can be substituted for more olive oil)
- ¼ cup beeswax pastilles
- 80 drops eucalyptus globulus essential oil
- 60 drops rosemary essential oil
- 60 drops white thyme essential oil (can be substituted with fir or cypress essential oil)
- 60 drops peppermint essential oil
- 40 drops lavender essential oil

DIRECTIONS

- In a double boiler combine beeswax and oils. Melt ingredients.
- Once ingredients are completely melted, remove from heat and add essential oils.
- Pour into containers to cool. Once cool, store in a dark cool area for maximum shelf life.

TO USE: Dab a small amount onto your fingers and apply generously to your chest, back, and feet to help open up airways and ease breathing. You can also use a small scoop of this in a cup of hot water to make a steam inhalant. Use as often as needed. A little bit goes a LONG way!

Aunt Flo's Soothing Salve

There has been one area of my life, that going natural and medicine free, has been a problem. That's during the time of the month that Aunt Flo decides to come out and visit. I have Endometriosis and Poly Cystic Ovarian Syndrome, and because of this, my periods are VERY painful. I am talking the kind of pain that has me curled up in a ball in bed, wishing it would just be over with already.

I was terrified to give up my use of Advil. I don't use it for anything else during the rest of the month, just for those first three days, when the pain is unbearable. Even just using it that small amount. once a month, was really starting to wear on my guilty conscience. I was terrified to give up my use of Advil. I don't use it for anything else during the rest of the month, just for those first three days, when the pain is unbearable. Even just using it that small amount. once a month, was really starting to wear on my guilty conscience.

Using this salve has been revolutionary for me and my monthly pains. I now combine this with a moon tea made with cramp bark and red raspberry leaf, and I no longer experience the extremely painful periods that I used to. In this recipe, I use the anti-inflammatory oil (from Chapter 10) that I also use in my Arnica Sore Muscle Salve, to help this salve really take care of all of my pains. I like to massage this on my abdomen, lower back, and thighs to relieve all of my aches and pains that come with Aunt Flo's visit.

INGREDEINTS

- ¾ cup olive oil (I like to use the anti-inflammatory oil from Chapter 10)
- ¼ cup beeswax pastilles
- 30 drops geranium essential oil
- 40 drops lavender essential oil
- 30 drops roman chamomile essential oil
- 40 drops clary sage essential oil
- 40 drops bergamot essential oil
- 60 drops clove essential oil
- 40 drops ginger essential oil
- 40 drops black pepper essential oil

DIRECTIONS

• Combine ingredients in a double boiler and melt. Remove from heat.

• Add essential oils and pour into tins or jars to store.

TO USE: Dab a small amount onto your fingers and massage onto the abdomen, lower back, and thighs. Use as often as needed.

Arnica Sore Muscle Salve

This salve is a miracle worker when it comes to sore muscles, bruises, aches, pains, and strains. My clientele even find a good deal of relief from arthritis with this salve. My personal massage therapist loves to use this salve while massaging me, both for my muscles and also for her hands. I use this salve for every ache and pain that I experience. It works even better when you add heat such as one of those bean bags that you put in the microwave to heat up.

INGREDEINTS

- ¾ cup olive oil (substitute the anti-inflammatory oil from Chapter 10, for best results)
- ¼ cup beeswax pastilles
- 60 drops peppermint essential oil
- 60 drops clove essential oil
- 40 drops lavender essential oil
- 40 drops eucalyptus globulus essential oil
- 40 drops rosemary essential oil
- 40 drops sweet marjoram essential oil
- 20 drops turmeric essential oil

DIRECTIONS

• Combine oil and beeswax in a double boiler and melt. Remove from heat.
• Add essential oils and pour into tins or jars to store.
TO USE: Dab a small amount onto your fingers and massage into sore and achy muscles. Use as often as needed.

Headcase Natural Headache Relief Roll-On

Headaches, migraines, and sinus pressure can really be a drag when we have a million things going on. The use of Tylenol, Advil, and other NSAIDs can be very damaging to your liver and all have many awful side effects. Certain essential oils have been proven to be effective in relieving headaches and migraines naturally, without all the nasty side effects!

I designed this roll-on to be an easy effective natural method of relieving headaches and migraines. My dad was one of the first people (outside of myself of course) to try out my headache roll-on, and though skeptical at first, he now shouts from the rooftops to anyone who will listen, about how effective this is.

Because some headaches are not stress related, but sinus related, I have added eucalyptus and chamomile essential oils to this to also aid in relieving sinus headaches. I also added sweet marjoram essential oil to aid in migraine and period headache relief. With this addition, this roll-on is also great to roll on your chest and toes to open up the airways and breathe easier.

INGREDIENTS

- 25 drops peppermint essential oil
- 25 drops lavender essential oil
- 5 drops roman chamomile essential oil
- 20 drops eucalyptus essential oil
- 15 drops sweet marjoram essential oil
- carrier oil to fill
- 1/3 oz. Roll-on bottle

DIRECTIONS

• Combine essential oils and carrier oil in a roll-on bottle. Shake to combine well.

TO USE: Gently shake the bottle before every use, to mix all oils together evenly. For headaches, roll on the back of your neck, on your temples, and if needed on the middle of your forehead between your eyebrows. (keep out of your eyes!) This also works very well to aid in sinus relief and opening up the airways. Just roll onto your chest and/or the bottoms of your toes/feet. Essential oils take anywhere from 15-35 minutes to enter the blood stream and begin working effectively. This roll-on usually takes about 15-20 minutes to reduce the pain of your headache/migraine, though for some this does work instantly!

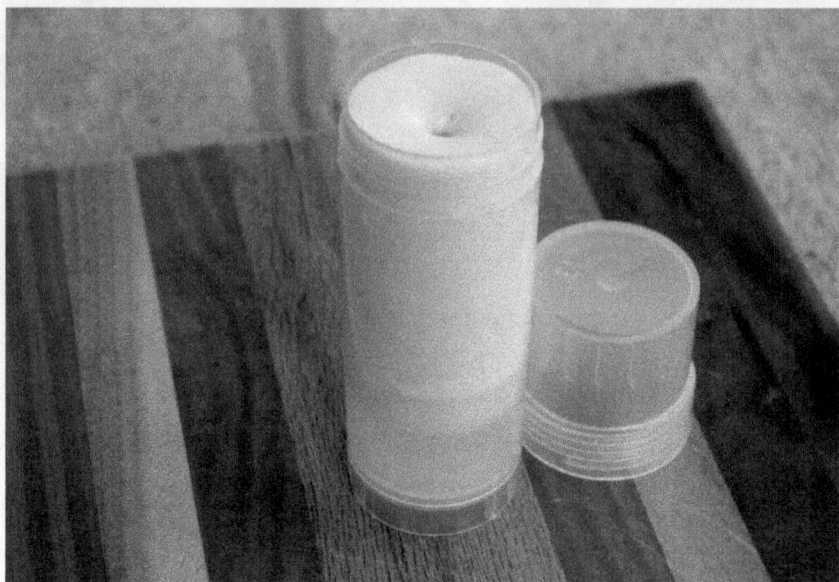

Sol Protection Sun Stick

Many conventional sunscreens sold at your local grocery and convenience stores contain toxic ingredients including endocrine disrupting chemicals, that experts say are changing us for the worst. Studies have shown that the use of these sunscreens may in fact promote skin cancer growth and free radical production. Since sunscreen's introduction into society, skin cancer rates haven't actually gone down. In fact, skin cancer rates have risen since the introduction of sunscreen and the FDA has even been caught saying "The FDA is not aware of data demonstrating that sunscreen use alone helps to prevent skin cancer".

Diet can improve the skin's resistance to the sun's harmful rays

Pretty much every illness that our body gets, is affected by what our body ingests, including our diet. Our skin is the largest organ in our body making it just as susceptible to a poor diet as any of our other organs. A diet that is low in antioxidants and high in over processed foods will make your skin much more susceptible to sun burns and damage. In general, fruits and vegetables are foods high in antioxidants and help us fight free radicals and sun damage, while foods such as meat, dairy products, simple carbohydrates, sugar and processed foods cause inflammation and can contribute to making our sun damage worse. Just by eating a whole foods diet that contains foods rich in antioxidants, you can help aid your skin's resistance to the sun's harmful rays. Some foods that have been known to help your body aid in sun protection are:

• Berries – strawberries, blueberries, raspberries, pomegranate, etc. – most berries are all extremely high in antioxidants and have been known to contain sun protecting properties in them. Makes sense since they are all ready for eating during the heat of the summer!
• Beans, nuts, legumes
• Green veggies

Sun protection via natural ingredients

Did you know that many of the unrefined butters and oils in your body butters and lotions, actually have natural sun protecting qualities? These are

• Raspberry seed oil - This is the most popular of oils to use for sun protection! Jam packed with a huge amount of antioxidants, raspberry seed oil has an estimated SPF of 28-50.
• Carrot seed essential oil - Carrot seed oil contains Carotenoids, which help decrease skin damage from UV radiation exposure. Carrots contain over 600 identified Carotenoids, making them an unparalleled source of antioxidants. Carrot seed oil has the highest concentration of Carotenoids available. Carrot seed oil has an estimated SPF of 38-40
• Wheat germ oil - This ultra nourishing oil has an SPF around 20
• Coconut oil - Coconut oil is a prized oil in skin care and hair care. It is used in everything from oil pulling to body butters. Coconut oil not only has antibacterial, anti-fungal, and anti-aging properties, but it also contains an SPF of roughly 5-10.
• Shea butter, Cocoa butter, Mango butter - All of these butters are great for your skin and help aid in repair and rejuvenation, but they also contain an SPF of 6-15
• Hemp seed oil, Avocado seed oil, Sunflower oil, Almond Oil - All great oils to deeply moisturize the skin as well as heal scars and lessen wrinkles, these oils also have SPF's that range from 5-15.
• Zinc oxide (non-nanoparticle) - a mineral that is created by oxidizing zinc. Zinc oxide provides full spectrum coverage from UVA and UVB long and short waves. Zinc oxide also has natural anti-inflammatory properties, making it a great addition to all sorts of healing creams on the market. Depending on the percentage you use of Zinc oxide, you can increase the amount of sun protection in your recipe.

INGREDEINTS

- 1/4 cup + 1 Tbsp. butter (I use 3 Tbsp. Shea butter, 1 Tbsp. mango butter, and 1 Tbsp. cocoa butter)
- 1/4 coconut oil
- 1 Tbsp. liquid oil (I use 1 tsp. raspberry seed oil, 1 tsp. hemp seed oil, and 1 tsp. avocado oil)
- 1/4 cup beeswax (If you want a harder consistency, use more beeswax, If you would like it softer add less. To make this as a body butter without the beeswax, just replace the beeswax with butters and whip as instructed in my body butter post)
- 2 Tbsp. non-nano zinc oxide (this can be adjusted based upon the SPF you are trying to achieve. I used roughly a 15% addition, see this chart here to adjust your recipe to your own needs.)
- 1 tsp. vitamin e
- essential oils (optional – I use 20 drops lavender, 10 drops carrot seed, 10 drops frankincense, and 5 drops roman chamomile. My essential oil blend is based on skin needs and not scent, you can use other essential oils to achieve specific scents but unless steam distilled, avoid citrus essential oils because they can cause skin sensitization which is brought about by sunlight!)

DIRECTIONS

•   In a double boiler melt butters, coconut oil, and beeswax. Once melted, continue to leave on heat for 20 minutes to process the butters.

•   After 20 minutes, remove from heat and stir in liquid oils and essential oils (if using)

•   Wearing a mask to cover your mouth/nose (or just your t-shirt covering you nose) mix in the zinc oxide. It is best not to breathe in the zinc oxide powder.

•   Whisk really well before pouring. I like to stir before each pour to be sure that the zinc oxide is mixed evenly. Pour into containers and store in a cool dark location when not in use. I use 2 oz. twist up tubes for easy application!

Sol Relief After Sun Spray

I have Greek skin, making me less prone to burning. Growing up, I never really put sunblock on because I usually just tanned instead of burning, and if it did burn, it easily turned brown by the next morning. My skin tone comes from my father, who also has less problems with burning. My mother, on the other hand could spend five minutes in the sun and burn her entire body. From her, I learned how to take care of a sunburn.

Many natural remedies for burns, have been around for centuries and are tried and true! In fact I created my Sol Relief spray based off of some of those old time remedies. I knew that I wanted to make a spray that was instantly cooling to the skin, to give instant relief, but also contained healing elements to prevent peeling and turn the burn into a tan. My Sol Relief spray does just that!

Home remedies for natural after-sun care

There are many natural remedies out there to help soothe and heal a nasty sunburn, and many of them can be found in your pantry or fridge!

•   Cold Water - Your first line of defense for burns, you should be running cold water onto your burn or take a cool bath to get the heat out of the skin. I remember way back in first-aid training, we were told that before application of any cream or aloe, that the burn needed to be fully cooled so that we didn't trap heat in, cooking the burn worse. A cool bath is easiest on a full body sunburn. You can add herbs, tea bags, sea salt, and/or oatmeal to your cooling bath to boost the soothing and healing powers.

•   Aloe Vera Gel - One of the most commonly used treatments for burns, aloe Vera is a powerhouse soother and healer. Keeping it in the fridge can up the awesome cooling powers of aloe too!

•   Coconut Oil - One of the best moisturizers out there, coconut oil can help heal any skin wound very quickly. Antibacterial and antiseptic, using coconut oil to keep the burn moisturized is key in avoiding peeling. Coconut oil is rich in antioxidants, fatty acids, and vitamins that promote healthy healing of burns.

•   Apple Cider Vinegar - This is a classic old timey remedy that really helps to stop the sting of the burn. Dip a washcloth into a mixture of apple cider vinegar and cold water, and apply to the burn to stop the pain and aid in quicker healing.

•   Peppermint Essential Oil - Not only is this essential oil antibacterial and antiseptic, but it also helps to aid in cooling the skin. I never leave this out of my after-sun sprays. The cooling effect can work for cooling down an overheated person too. The trick is to spray the back of the neck and the bottoms of the feet.

- Lavender Essential Oil - Lavender essential oil is said to have many amazing healing benefits when it comes to skin and burns. Not only is it an analgesic, helping to relieve pain, but lavender is also able to regenerate cell tissue and minimize scarring. This all-purpose essential oil has been used for centuries to heal, but its burn-healing abilities were first recorded in 1907 by a French Chemist, Dr. René-Maurice Gattefossé. After burning his badly during one of his experiments, he dunked it in the nearest vat of liquid, which happened to be lavender essential oil. After watching in amazement how quickly his burn healed, and with minimal scarring, he began studying and writing about essential oils further.
- Colloidal Silver - Used in burn centers all across the country as a natural and effective treatment, when nothing else will heal a burn, colloidal silver is a natural antibiotic that has been used for centuries to build immunities, heal skin wounds, and help cure the common cold. I even put drops of colloidal silver in my kiddo's ears to help heal and prevent ear infections.
- Raw Honey - Used by holistic Doctors and Veterinarians alike, honey is used as a natural ointment for all kinds of owies, including burns. Naturally antibacterial and antiseptic, raw honey has been clinically proven to support wound healing faster and better than Neosporin.
- Black or Green Tea - Naturally rich in tannins, the tannic acid helps to suck out the heat of the burn, therefore alleviating the pain! You can take a refreshing cold tea bath, or just make a big batch of iced tea and soak washcloths in it and cover the burn. Allow the tea to air dry on your skin. Repeat this 3 times a day until the burn is healed.
- Plantain - This plant is often thought of as a weed in North America but has been hailed by not only the Native Americans but also Alexander the great, for being a miracle worker with burns, bug bites, and stings. A strong infusion of plantain sprayed onto a sunburn as often as needed can help soothe a sunburn and heal it faster. Plantain contains a compound called allatonin, an anti-inflammatory phytochemical that speeds wound healing, stimulates the grow of new skin cells, and gives the immune system a boost.
- Sea Salt - Like baking soda, sea salt can help to get rid of the sting and relieve pain and soreness from the burn. Add 1/4-1/2 cup of salt to your bath. Don't soak for longer than 20-30 minutes as this can dry out your burn too much. Pat your body dry and gently apply aloe Vera and/or coconut oil to your burn.

• Calendula Tincture or Tea - Calendula is very effective at healing many different skin conditions. You can use the herb to make a tincture or a strong tea, and apply it to the burn in a cold compress. If you don't have a tincture on hand add a drop to water)hen you get burned, just make a strong infusion and apply the tea to the burn a couple of hours. You can soak a cloth in the tea and wrap it around the burn if needed.

• Egg Whites - There is no telling where this remedy came from. I've seen it floating all over the internet, but I will say that it does in fact work. Not only have I read of many other people who have found this odd remedy to soothe their pain, I too have used this on a burn on my hand that the oven gave me. Just separate the whites from the yolks and apply to sunburn. It will help to cool the burn and ease the pain.

• Baking Soda - Baking soda added to a cool bath is great at reliving pain and soreness from a nasty burn. Just add a 1/4-1/2 cup to your bath and submerse your burn. Don't do this for longer than 20-30 minutes, to prevent over drying your burn. Pat your body dry and gently apply aloe and/or coconut oil to your sunburn.

• Oatmeal Bath - I make a really great oatmeal bath that I sell in my Etsy Shoppe. You can always make your own oatmeal bath from a recipe I shared awhile back too! Oatmeal baths are great for relieving all sorts of skin irritations including sunburns! Combine oatmeal and baking soda with some essential oils for the ultimate sunburn relief bath.

INGREDEINTS

- 6 Tbsp. peppermint hydrosol (optional – this can be replaced with more water, but it is what gives this spray the extra cooling effect!)
- 4 Tbsp. aloe Vera gel
- 1/2 Tbsp. vegetable glycerin (optional - helps give extra moisture to the skin to heal the burn faster)
- 1 Tbsp. apple cider vinegar (I use apple cider vinegar that I have steep in dried peppermint leaf and sage leaf)
- 1/2 Tbsp. colloidal silver (optional - this is used all over the world in vet offices and some doctor's offices to help heal many different skin conditions and abrasions. It helps to keep the wound clean and acts as a natural antibiotic to help prevent infection)
- 10 drops peppermint essential oil
- 10 drops lavender essential oil

- distilled water to fill
- 8 oz. spray bottle

DIRECTIONS

• Combine ingredients in spray bottle, cap, and shake well before use.

TO USE: Spray as often as needed, onto burned or sun-exposed skin for cooling and moisturizing relief. Avoid spraying eyes! Refrigerate for an even more soothing and cooling experience and to keep the product longer.

Anti-Itch Calamine Lotion

When I was a little girl, I used to romp around with my little sister all over my grandparents farm in California. My grandmother would push us out the back door in the morning and tell us not to come back until lunch time. Whenever we inevitably got ourselves into a scrape, she always had just the right remedy in her pantry, to fix the problem. This recipe is great for all sorts of itch relief. Bug bites, chicken pox, poison ivy and oak, and more!

INGREDEINTS

- 1 Tbps. sea salt
- 1 Tbsp. baking soda
- 1 Tbsp. bentonite clay (remember not to use any metal when using bentonite clay, as this will react with the clay making it less effective.)
- water/witch hazel to form a paste (I often use witch hazel for its astringent properties as well as its ability to help relieve itching.)
- 5 drops lavender essential oil (*optional* - highly antibacterial, anti-inflammatory, and analgesic)
- 5 drops peppermint essential oil (*optional* - helps reduce itchiness and inflammation)
- 5 drop chamomile essential oil (*optional* - helps reduce inflammation and is a natural antihistamine)

DIRECTIONS

• Combine all of the dry ingredients in a small bowl.

- Slowly add in the water/witch hazel until a smooth and creamy paste forms, then add in the essential oils if using.
- Apply to itchy bug bites, chicken pox, rashes, and more!

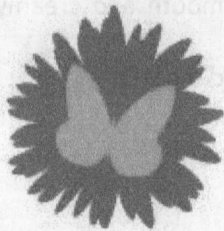

Chapter 6

Hippy Dudes

Guys can be very simplistic with their cosmetic needs. It's obvious that most of us women take up the most space on the bathroom counters, but there are still things that every guy buys, that you can make for yourself at home. With a husband who loves his beard and a dad who loves to keep it clean shaven, I have my own guinea pigs at my disposal to test all of my recipes out. They are big fans of all the products I give them! In fact many of my male clients rave about their soft beards and smooth skin.

Hairy Hippy Beard Oil

My Husband is a bearded man. He has had his beard the entire that I have known him, and the very few times he shaved it off...he did not look right to me at all. I used to think that beards weren't attractive, and yet now I'd miss his beard terribly, if he shaved it off. I designed this beard oil to help soften and smooth his beard hair so that it would stop prickling my lips. No one likes to kiss a prickly beard!

Manly Essential Oil Blends For Beard Oil

10 drops rosemary

5 drops lavender

5 drops white thyme

10 drops lemon

5 drops patchouli

3 drops cardamom

3 drops cedarwood

10 drops bergamot

10 drops cedarwood

10 drops clove

3 drops lime

5 drops nutmeg

2 drops vanilla absolute

3 drops bay

3 drops pine

10 drops rosemary

3 drops juniper berry

10 drops cedarwood

10 drops sweet orange

3 drops nutmeg

5 drops clove

INGREDEINTS

- 1 oz. glass bottle with dropper
- 1 Tbsp. base carrier oil (this can be almond oil, avocado oil, grapeseed oil, hemp seed oil or any combination thereof)
- 1/2 Tbsp. jojoba oil
- 1/2 Tbsp. extra special carrier oil (you can either substitute this for more jojoba or add in some argan oil, rosehip seed oil, pumpkin seed oil etc.)
- essential oil blend

DIRECTIONS

• Combine all ingredients in glass bottle with a dropper top and label for the hairy hippy in your life!

• When using, put 5-8 drops (depending on beard size) of moisturizing beard oil in the palm of your hand and massage into your beard and onto your face.

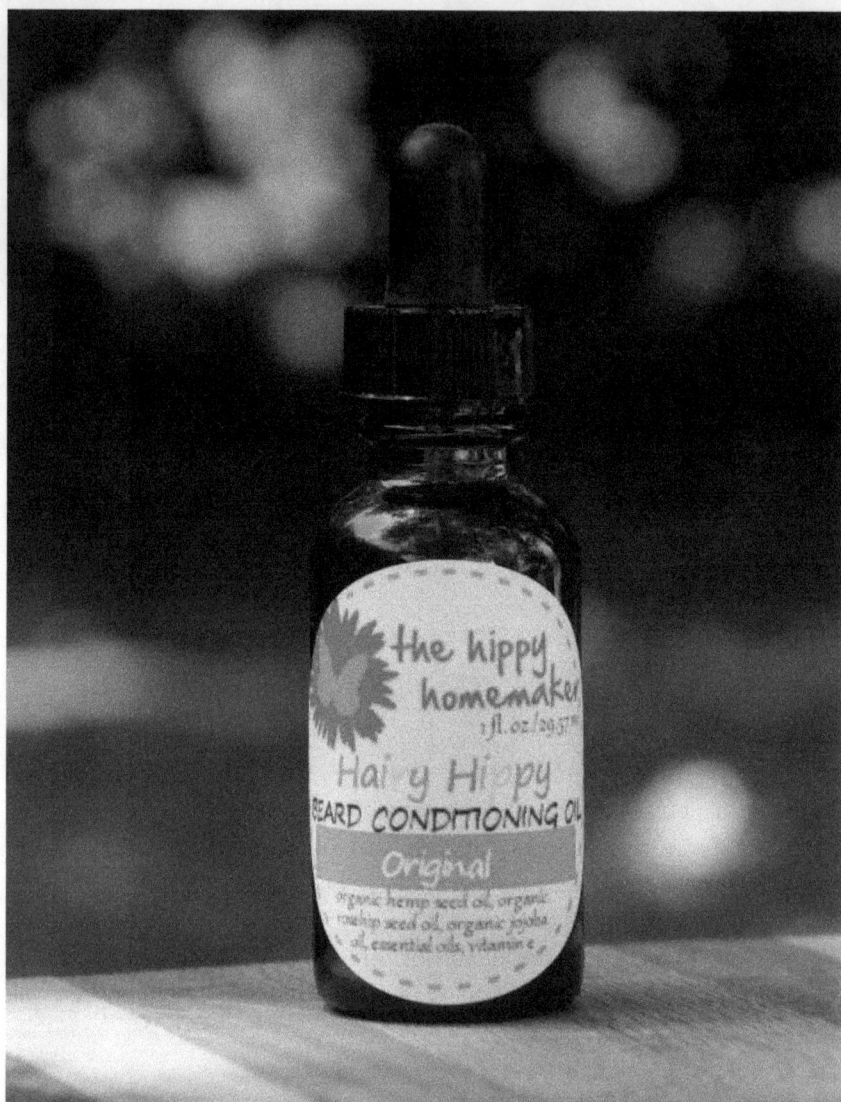

Hairless Hippy Aftershave

After shaving with your homemade shaving cream from Chapter 4, an after shave is essential to helping close the pores and moisturize the skin for a clean cut shave that feels smooth and soft to the touch.

INGREDEINTS

- 4 oz. Spray bottle
- ¼ cup witch hazel

- 1 Tbsp. Aloe Vera gel (*optional* – but really helps to moisturize and heal the skin)
- 1 tsp. Vegetable glycerin (*optional* – but really helps to moisturize the skin)
- 1 tsp. Colloidal silver (*optional* – not only does this help heal and soothe red inflamed skin, colloidal silver is known to help prevent razor burn too!)
- water or hydrosol to fill
- 20 drops lavender essential oil
- 10 drops cedarwood essential oil
- 10 drops cypress essential oil

DIRECTIONS

• Combine ingredients in 4 oz. spray bottle and shake to combine.

FOR USE: Spray on freshly shaven face and either air dry or pat dry with a towel.

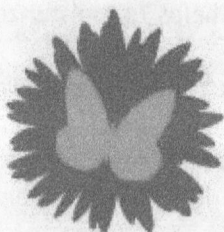

Chapter 7

Lip Care & Make-Up

Makeup has pretty much been around since the dawn of man-kind. Used during ceremonies, plays, ritual, for beauty, and more, the practice of using our bodies as our canvas for our own art, has been a staple for all civilizations. Cleopatra was well known to love the use of many different types of cosmetics. From the use of lip stains to eye liners, Cleopatra had the best natural ingredients at her disposal. Using the supplies that are found around your home, you can pretty much make most of your glamor products at home yourself. The best part is that you can customize your cosmetics to match your skin tones and lip colors to your needs!

Hippy Lippy Lip Balms

One of the first things that I learned how to make for myself was lip balms. I was so excited at how easy it was to make a decent lip balm, I decided to make everyone homemade lip balms for Christmas that year. I got such rave reviews from everyone, over how awesome the lip balms were, I began making more for sale.

You can make this a red/pink tinted lip balm by first steeping the oils in this recipe, in either beet root powder, alkanet root powder, or hibiscus flowers. After straining the coloring herbs out of the oils, proceed with melting the beeswax and butters.

The essential oils can be replaced with other essential oils and/or flavor extracts. Be sure to use caution with your essential oil choices for lip balms.

INGREDEINTS

- 2 Tbsp. Coconut oil
- 2 – 2 ½ Tbsp. Beeswax (I use 2 in the wintertime and 2 ½ during the hot Texas summertime)

- 1 Tbsp. Butter (Shea butter, mango butter, cocoa butter, or kokum butter are all great options here)
- ½ Tbsp. Liquid carrier oil (I use hemp seed but you can use any number of liquid oils here!)

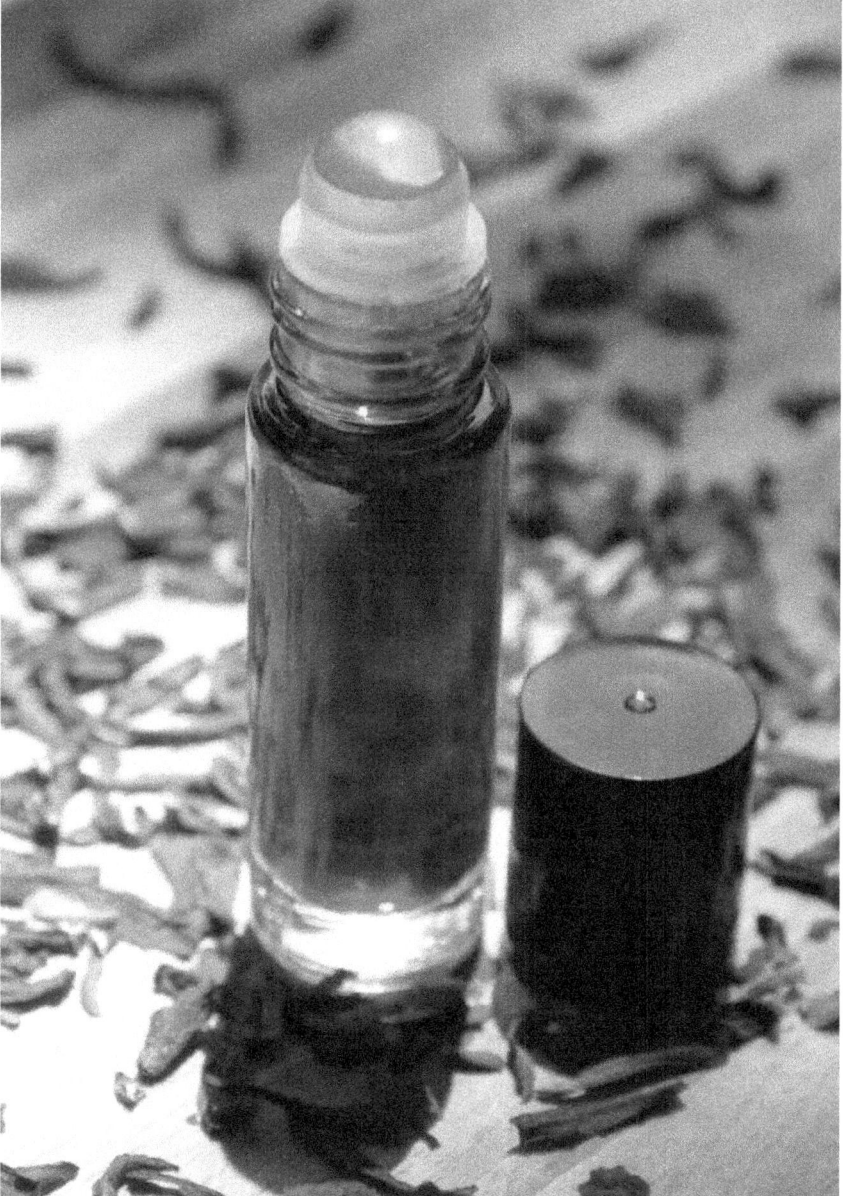

- ½ Tbsp. Castor oil (or more liquid carrier oil. Castor oil is the perfect addition to lip balms because of it gives just a tad bit of shine to the lip balm as well as provides a large amount of moisturization for really dry and peeling lips)

- ½ tsp. Vitamin e (*optional*)
- 30 drops peppermint essential oil
- 25 drops lavender essential oil

DIRECTIONS

• In a double boiler, melt coconut oil, butter, and beeswax. Once melted, allow to remain on the heat for 20 minutes to process the butters.

• Remove from heat and add liquid oils, vitamin e, and essential oils/flavor oils. Pour into lip balm tubes and allow to cool and harden.

Lip Stains

The earliest known evidence of the use of lip color was in ancient Mesopotamia, where the use of crushed semi-precocious stones were applied to the lips to stimulate color. Cleopatra was known for her bright red lip stain, extracted from the juices of crushed beetles. The ancient Egyptians were even known to use henna to stain their lips. There are many items you can choose to use, including herbs and fruits, to make a great lip stain.

Berry Berry Lip & Cheek Stain

INGREDEINTS

- raspberries
- black berries
- pomegranate seeds
- extra virgin olive oil

DIRECTIONS

• Mash up all the berries and pomegranate seeds until you have released all of the juices.

• Strain the juice/mash through a sieve and squeeze all of the juices out.

• Add a couple drops of olive oil and store in an airtight container in your fridge for up to 1 week.

- Using your finger, apply to lips and let dry. Doing this several times can layer darker and darker color to your lips. Apply an oil based lip balm or gloss when dry. This also doubles as a cheek stain!

Cosmic Crush Hibiscus Lip Stain

This is the lip stain that I sell in my shoppe and my clients are in LOVE with it! Made with only 3 ingredients, this lip stain is vegan and extremely easy to make, though it does take some time for the hibiscus extract to steep, beyond that, this recipe is very simple! All you need is a 1/3 oz. roll on bottle.

INGREDEINTS

- 2 Tbsp. Dried hibiscus flowers (you can alternately make this with beet root powder or alkanet root powder)
- 1 cup 80 proof (or higher) vodka
- vegetable glycerin

DIRECTIONS

- In a mason jar combine hibiscus and vodka. Allow to steep for 2 weeks, shaking once or twice a day. Strain and store hibiscus extract in a cool dark place.
- In a 1/3 oz. roll on bottle, fill it ¾ of the way with hibiscus extract. Fill the remaining ¼ of the bottle with vegetable glycerin. Cap and shake until well combined.

TO USE: Use on clean dry lips. If color is splotchy, exfoliate lips to achieve a smoother look! To use, roll onto lips and let completely dry before applying and oil based gloss or lip balm to add shine. The color can be applied in layers to achieve desired hue.

Honey & Cinnamon Lip Scrub

Don't shell out big bucks for suspect ingredients. When I go shopping around the internet for any one of the supposed "high end" products like Sephora's lip scrub and Bliss's Fabulips, I find that you end up shelling out $20-$25 for a half ounce of product that contains many suspect ingredients in them. I don't know about you, but I don't really want to put stuff on my lips that contain ingredients that could be carcinogenic or cause allergic reactions (such as fragrances). Not to mention that fact that anything going on your lips could accidentally be ingested through your mouth as well! For a quarter of the price, you can make eight times as much lip scrub, and know that you are getting the highest quality product. Honey is naturally healing to the body and the skin. Did you know that many veterinarians use organic raw unfiltered honey as a natural owie cream? It's natural antibiotic and antiviral properties are so wonderful that just a dab of it on a cut or scrape can help it to heal fast.

INGREDEINTS

- 1/4 cup brown sugar (you can use regular sugar here or even salt but brown sugar is tastier!)
- 1 Tbsp. coconut oil (this can be substituted with any sort of oil such as almond, olive, etc.)
- 1 Tbsp. raw unfiltered honey
- 1 tsp. cinnamon powder (you can even do ginger powder, nutmeg, or cloves.)

DIRECTIONS

•   Combine ingredients in a small bowl and transfer to a small jar with a lid.

TO USE: Rub a small amount onto your lips in a circular motion for 1-2 minutes. Rinse (or you could just lick it off if you really wanted too....) off with a wet washcloth and feel the difference! Follow with an oil based lip balm to lock in moisture!

Natural Black Mascara and Eye Liner

I have blonde tipped eye lashes. If I could only choose one makeup item to beautify my face, it would definitely be mascara. This natural mascara is not waterproof, but it does have pretty good staying power. It won't melt off of your lashes in the heat like some of the ones that require oils and butters to create, which is why this is my favorite recipe.

INGREDEINTS

- 2 tsp. pure aloe Vera gel
- 10 capsules activated charcoal, opened and emptied. To open the capsules, simply twist the two halves and gently pull them apart.
- A little less than ¼ tsp clay (white clay or bentonite clay both are great options)

- an empty (clean and sterilized) mascara container (you can also store this in a small glass jar, just be sure it seals properly because this will dry out otherwise)

DIRECTIONS

• Mix all of the ingredients together until smooth and consistent.
• To fill the tube, use an oral syringe these can be purchased at the drugstore for a few dollars and will make the process significantly more simple). Fill the syringe, then transfer the mixture into the mascara tube by pushing the plunger. Wipe off any excess mixture.
• Apply mascara in coats, allowing each coat to dry for a minute before adding another. Use an eyelash comb or clean mascara wand to brush out any clumps.

Powdered Blush

I just love how easy this recipe is to make! This recipe can either be kept as loose blush or compacted down into a recycled compact container. You could theoretically dried fruit powders as well as dried herb powders to get the color blush you are trying to attain. Add more or less arrowroot powder to custom create the color you are looking for. Some herb and fruit variations that would make lovely blush colors are hibiscus, beet root, alkanet root, ginger root, turmeric, dried raspberries, dried strawberries, dried bananas, cocoa powder, rosehips, dried carrots.

INGREDEINTS

- 4 tsp. Color powder
- 1-2 tsp. Arrowroot powder

DIRECTIONS

• Combine color powder and arrowroot powder until desired color is achieved.
• This can either be packed into an old powder container, or kept loose for application. I like to add about one drop of lavender essential oil to this, to help pack it into my powder container.

Face Powder

Just like blush, this can be easily customize to achieve your own skin tone. Using different ratios of cocoa powder, arrowroot powder, cinnamon, and/or ginger, you can create a whole rainbow of skin tones.

INGREDEINTS

- cocoa powder
- cinnamon powder/ginger powder, (optional helps achieve some darker colors)
- 2 Tbsp. cornstarch or arrowroot powder

DIRECTIONS

•   Combine small amounts of cocoa (and cinnamon if you don't have sensitive skin) powder into 2 Tbsp. cornstarch (or arrowroot powder) until you find the right color for your skin type.

•   This can either be packed into an old powder container, or kept loose for application. I like to add about one drop of lavender essential oil to this to help pack it into my powder container.

Bronzer

Only in the wintertime do I need a bronzer. I was blessed with skin that instantly tans with any time spent out in the sun. Not everyone is as lucky as me, at getting that sun-kissed glow. This dry recipe can be whipped into the homemade body butter or lotion from chapter four. I love to make whipped bronzer butter!

INGREDEINTS

- 1 Tbsp. Cocoa powder (the
- ½ tsp. Cinnamon
- 1-2 tsp. Arrowroot powder

DIRECTIONS

•   Combine ingredients in a jar. Dust onto skin with a large powder brush. If wanting a bronzing lotion, combine with body butter or lotion from chapter 4 and apply bronzing lotion to skin and rub in. Allow to dry before dressing. Avoid wearing white with bronzing lotion.

Natural Homemade Foundation

A good natural foundation should be able to even out skin tone and splotchy marks, moisturize and keep healthy your skin, as well as give a bit of protection from UV rays. I designed this foundation to be able to do all three of these things without clogging your pores. This is best applied with a foundation applicator sponge, though it can be applied with your fingers if need be. This foundation is a light foundation and it not meant to be thickly applied.

SKIN TONE

- Light Foundation – ½ Tbsp. Cocoa powder
- Light to Medium Foundation – ½ Tbsp. + 1 tsp. Cocoa powder
- Medium to Dark Foundation – ½ Tbsp. + 2 tsp. Cocoa powder
- Dark Foundation 1 ½ Tbsp.+ cocoa powder

INGREDEINTS

- 3 Tbsp. Carrier oil (hemp seed is my favorite oil to use because it's considered a dry oil and will sink into the skin fairly quickly. This oil is great for all skin types including those with acne/oily skin types.)
- 2 Tbsp. Shea butter
- 1 Tbsp. Cocoa butter
- 1 Tbsp. Beeswax
- ¼ tsp. Vitamin e
- 1-2 Tbsp. Uncoated, non-nano, and non-microionized zinc oxide powder
- cocoa powder
- 1/8 tsp. Cinnamon powder

DIRECTIONS

- In a double boiler melt the beeswax, Shea butter, and cocoa cocoa butter. Let sit on the heat for 20 minutes to process the butters.
- Remove from heat. Add carrier oil and vitamin e. Wearing a mask, vigorously whisk in the zinc oxide, cocoa cocoa powder, and cinnamon powder.
- You can either whisk and pour this into jars or tins to cool; or you can take this one step further and create a whipped foundation by whipping this like you do with whipped body butter.
- Pour the entire concoction into a bowl and put the bowl into an ice bath to cool quicker.

- When it looks like the mixture is half way hardened, meaning there is still a small pool of liquid on top, take out your electric hand mixer or emulsion blender and start whipping the mixture until it's light and fluffy.
- If you blended too soon, don't fret, just leave the mixture be for another couple minutes in the ice bath and then blend while it's in the ice bath. I find that whipping the foundation like this makes this the best texture for the best application.

Easy Makeup Remover

I once used a makeup remover from one of the most popular brands on the market, that left me with intensely burning eyes! I had been trying to remove my eye makeup, in the same fashion that I always had, and a small amount of the eye makeup remover got into my eyes and started burning like I had gotten soap into them! It was a horrible experience, needless to say, and after learning just how easy it is to remove makeup at home, I will never have to buy a makeup remover again.

INGREDIENTS

- coconut oil

DIRECTIONS

- Using a soft washcloth, dab a very small amount of coconut oil onto your eyes and wipe makeup away. It's seriously that easy AND it will help moisturize the skin around your eyes to keep them wrinkle free!

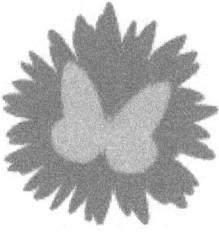

Chapter 8

Natural Hair Care

Before my hippy makeover was complete, I had made use of my teens and twenties to utterly destroy my hair. I dyed my hair pretty much every color of the rainbow, and back again. I used all sorts of flat irons, curling irons, crimpers, blow dryers (which is the one thing I still use periodically), etc. I tried ALL kinds of products containing harmful and harsh ingredients. All of this damage really started to stack up and my hair just became so dead that I really could never grow it out. I don't remember a time in my life that I had ever had hair passed my shoulders. It was so dry and brittle that I always had to keep it cut in cute bobs just to get rid of all the damage. I wasn't sure that I would ever know what my natural hair looked like, let alone see it look as sleek and smooth as some of those really lucky celebrities. Little did I know, with using the no-poo method, I could actually attain hair that I had figured was unattainable.

What is the no-poo method, you ask?

Unlike the sound of the name, no-pooing doesn't actually mean that you don't wash your hair. It seems to be a common misconception among many of the people that I have told about my hair washing regime. Most have asked me "doesn't your hair start to stink?" The answer to that is a resounding "no!" I am still washing my hair, I just choose to use something other than shampoo to get it clean.

The no-poo method is simply a method of washing one's hair with various ingredients other than shampoo, which usually contains SLS (Sodium Laurel Sulfate, a known carcinogen and is harmful to the environment). If you search the internet, you will find a plethora of differing recipes but the main ingredients in 90% of these recipes are baking soda and apple cider vinegar. Always a two step process, these recipes ask you to apply the baking soda to your hair, (sometimes in a paste form, other times in a spray/rinse form) rinse, then apply the diluted apple cider vinegar to your hair, and rinse again.

Detox takes time...sometimes a looonng time

The most difficult part of switching over to a no-poo lifestyle, is being patient while your scalp has a chance to catch up with the changes that you are making. This so-called detox period is filled with very greasy, stringy hair that feels heavy and oily. I had to put my hair up during my entire detox period because my hair was so greasy. For some people with already healthy hair, they may only experience a minimal two week detox with very little hair issues. For others, like myself, with a lot of hair damage, it can take up to three months to find the right balance. Once your hair finally finds the balance and adjusts to your new hair regime, it is advised not to let your hair stylist convince you to try the newest paraben-free shampoo she got in last week. You will have to detox all over again. Take it from someone who has had to experience this!

Why you should change what you're washing your hair with

Most conventional shampoos and conditioners that you find at your every day store, contain harsh toxic ingredients that is not only bad for your hair and scalp, but also bad for the environment too.

All of the toxic chemicals aside (we ALWAYS seem to be talking about them), there is another reason to be switching from commercial shampoos. Most commercial shampoos strip the scalp of its natural oils. This then leads your scalp to kick into gear and produce even more oils, making your hair oily if you don't wash it every day or two. Once you manage to get passed the detox period of no-pooing, you only need to wash your hair once or twice a week, if that. It sounds gross, but think about it from this angle; people didn't need to wash their hair daily or even every other day until the introduction of commercial detergents into shampoos.

My hair began falling out in clumps because of baking soda

I had read that a two week (even up to two months or more) detox period could be expected when trying to shed your hair of all of the build up of lab-created silicons, but after reading all of the benefits, I was still curious to see if I truly could find my naturally beautiful hair underneath all of this mess. There was no "at first my hair was amazingly soft and beautiful" like most of the blogs that I had read. I had destroyed my hair prior to this, so shedding all of the silicons that coated my hair just proved to show me how badly my hair was lacking in moisture.

The oils on my head began over producing big time and all I could do was put my hair up in a bun. I kept waiting for the moment when combing my hair in the shower didn't mean the loss of such precious strands by the dozen, but instead my hair-loss began to get worse. The Hippy Hubby even commented on how much hair was beginning to clog up the drain, and most of it was mine.

After two months of trying the no-poo method, I realized that it was not working out, but I couldn't figure out why. I knew that my hair was already damaged and it would take awhile to fix, but I figured that I would at least see improvement in my hair in a two month period of time. I decided it was time to go on a learning adventure and find out WHY I was having these problems.

PH is the key to balancing your hair and scalp

It turned out, my dry brittle hair was falling out due to the high alkalinity (PH) of the baking soda. After much research, I found that the key to balancing your hair and scalp starts with balancing the pH of the sebum on your scalp.

PH (Potential of Hydrogen) is the measure of alkalinity or acidity in a substance. PH can range anywhere from 1 (highly acidic) to 14 (highly alkaline). Human hair and skin has a layer of salt/water/oil that is called the acid mantle. This wonderfully protective layer lives happily at a PH of 4.5 and is easily disrupted and washed away with anything that has a pH over 7 (neutral and the pH of water).

Low quality hair care products can disrupt the pH of the hair. The pH of your hair dictates the health of it. If your haircare routine is to alkali, then your cuticles will stay open and your hair will be dry and brittle. If your haircare routine is one closer to the pH of hair, your hair's cuticles will be closed properly and your hair will be silky smooth and soft.

Learning about this put me on a deeper investigation to learn about PH and our hair. I discovered that though diluting baking soda can cause its PH to go down, it takes 20 cups of water to 1 Tbsp. of baking soda to make a pH of 9. That's way to alkaline for our hair and will cause it to be extremely dry and brittle, breaking off everywhere.

Using highly alkaline solutions on your hair such as baking soda or castile soap, though it feels soft and manageable, the disulfide bonds in your hair's internal structure is being weakened. Following this alkaline solution with an acidic solution to bring the pH back down is called clarifying. It can sometimes be OK for your hair and scalp once a month, but weekly clarifying is damaging to your hair.

What can you use to no-poo cleanse your hair?

With so much information out there purporting the awesomeness of the baking soda no-poo method, it leads one to wonder if there are any other options, but BEHOLD! There are actually quite a few options that you can wash your hair with, no-poo style. I have made a point of trying all of them for the sake of doing my research for you guys. (I might have also forced my husband to be a guinea pig along with me. I am really thankful that the Hippy Hubby allows me to use him for testing purposes!)

•   Aloe Vera – with a pH of 4.5-5.5, aloe Vera is a really great option to no-poo with. Combining equal parts aloe Vera gel and coconut milk in a blender, makes a divine no-poo.
•   Honey – with a pH of around 4, honey is also very conditioning to the hair and can help reduce frizz too! It makes a great conditioning addition to any no-poo recipe.
•   Apple Cider Vinegar – With a pH of 3-3.5 ACV is a great choice when diluted. I like to dilute mine with aloe Vera and water. Note that ACV is chosen over white vinegar because it has a higher pH than white vinegar.
•   Water – There are some people who simply just wash their hair with water. My own hair needs a lot more help than just water. I suspect this works on those who A) haven't really damage their hair any before the change AND B) have clean water that isn't too hard. Hard water can make a huge difference on how clean your hair gets, and it especially interacts with natural soaps like castile soap, leaving too much build up.
•   Herbal Infused Tea – There are so many hair healing herbs that you can use in some capacity in any natural no-poo method that you choose, but plain herbal tea can be used to cleanse and/or rinse your hair as well. See below for specific herbs to helps your hair type. I have seen great success with just herbal tea for my shampoo.

• Clay – Both Bentonite and Rhassoul clay have wonderful healing benefits, no only for our faces, but also for our hair! Containing a plethora of minerals and awesome cleansing powers, clay should not be ignored when making your own no-poo shampoo. Clay has the power to both cleanse and condition while keeping your scalp and hair's oil cycle in tact. (The pH of 1 Tbsp. Rhassoul clay and 8 oz. water can be a little high at 6, so it's always best to either add lower pH ingredients such as ACV or aloe Vera to the mix, or rinse with an apple cider vinegar rinse after washing.)

• Saponin Cleansing Herbs – Did you know that you can wash your hair with herbs that act like soap and get a little sudsy? If you have ever used soap nuts in your laundry to clean your clothes, then you have had a saponin cleansing herb all along! Saponins are plant versions of cleansing suds and can be used in place of soap to clean things including our hair! Saponin cleansing herbs include yucca root, soapnuts, and soapwort.

Hair healing herbs for health and growth

There are so many great herbs to use in your hair recipes! Whether you have dry hair, oily hair, thinning hair, or even want a color boost, you can use herbs to help you make your hair healthier and happier!

Normal hair: Basil, Calendula, Chamomile, Horsetail, Lavender, Linden flowers, Nettle, Parsley leaf, Rosemary, Sage, Watercress

Dry hair and scalp: Burdock root, Calendula, Chamomile, Comfrey leaf, Elder flowers, Horsetail, Lavender, Marshmallow root, Nettle, Parsley leaf, Sage

Oily hair and scalp: Bay leaf, Burdock root, Calendula, Chamomile, Horsetail, Lemon Balm, Lavender, Lemon peel, Lemongrass, Nettle, Peppermint, Rosemary, Thyme, Witch Hazel bark, Yarrow leaf and flower

Scalp conditions (dandruff, sensitive skin, inflammation, itchiness, dermatitis): Burdock root, Calendula, Chamomile, Comfrey leaf, Eucalyptus, Horsetail, Lavender, Marshmallow root, Nettle, Oregano, Peppermint, Rosemary, Sage, Thyme

Hair loss/thinning: Basil, Nettle, Rosemary, Sage

Golden highlights: Calendula, Chamomile, Lemon, Sunflower petals

Dark highlights: Black Tea, Black Walnut hulls (crushed or chopped),

Comfrey root, Nettle, Rosemary, Sage

Red highlights: Calendula, Henna, Hibiscus flowers, Red Clover flowers, Rose hips, Red Rose petals

Silken Goddess Apple Cider Vinegar Rinse

This hair conditioning rinse is what I use for pretty much everything. When I need a leave-in conditioning detangler, I go to this spray. When I am out of homemade shampoo, I wash with this. When I need to refresh my curls with my diffusor, I just wet my hair with this rinse. After every no-poo and henna treatment I follow with this apple cider vinegar rinse. It is one of my most important ingredients in my natural hair care regime. I usually steep my apple cider vinegar in hair healing herbs (such as marshmallow root, oatstraw, horsetail, nettle, green tea, etc.) for two weeks, before using in this recipe.

INGREDEINTS

- 16 oz spray bottle
- 2 Tbsp. Apple cider vinegar
- 2 Tbsp. Aloe Vera gel
- water to fill
- 20 drops essential oils (I like to use peppermint sage, lavender, grapefruit lavender, and lime and vanilla in my spray bottle)

DIRECTIONS

• Combine ingredients in a spray bottle. Spray directly onto hair. Does not have to be rinsed from hair, as the mild vinegar scent dissipates as it dries!

Herbal Goddess Shampoo

This shampoo is so amazing, I still can't believe how soft it makes my hair. I am most shocked by the fact that I use no actual soap in the recipe, but saponin filled herbs and nourishing ingredients. This recipe is my go to no-poo in my shower!

INGREDEINTS

- 2 cups distilled water/hydrosol (I love to replace the water in this recipe with hydrosol, coconut milk, or aloe Vera juice)
- 2-3 Tbsp. Soapwort

- 1-2 whole soap nuts
- 1 Tbsp. Marshmallow root
- 1 Tbsp. Horsetail
- 1 Tbsp. Oatstraw
- 1 Tbsp. Hibiscus (this can be replaced with chamomile, lavender, calendula, etc.)
- ¼ cup apple cider vinegar (I like to infuse mine with herbs that are great for my hair like marshmallow root, horsetail, green tea, etc.)
- ¼ cup aloe Vera gel
- 1 tsp. Guar gum powder
- ½ tsp. Citric acid
- colloidal silver (*optional* – I add this to all of my hair recipes because it not only helps with hair growth and healing but is a known anti-fungal and can be used in conjunction with citric acid to provide a small amount of preservation.)
- 20 drops essential oils (I like to use peppermint sage, grapefruit lavender, or chamomile rose as some of the mixtures that I do. Always research the essential oils that you choose to use in your body care products.)

DIRECTIONS

• Combine distilled water, soapwort, soap nuts, and marshmallow root in a small pan. Bring to a boil and turn heat down to simmer for 20 minutes.

• Remove from heat and add horsetail, oatstraw, and any other herbs you might be steeping. Leave to steep until the liquid is cool. Strain herbs from the liquid with a mesh strainer or cheese cloth. Stir in citric acid until dissolved.

• Combine tea liquid with apple cider vinegar, aloe Vera juice, and colloidal silver. Using a whisk, whisk in guar gum powder until dissolved into the shampoo and is thickened. If adding essential oils, whisk in now too.

TO USE: Pour a sufficient amount into your wetted hair and massage into your hair as you would soap shampoos. Let sit in your hair for five minutes, rinse. If needed, you can follow with the apple cider vinegar rinse.

The Hippy Homemaker's Ultra Awesome Hair Cleansing and Conditioning Mud

I found only a small hand full of products that follow the no-poo style of cleansing the hair, and those few products can be a bit pricey for some. My hair cleansing mud has proven to be the BEST thing I have ever felt on my hair..EVER. Seriously, the moment I rinsed the mud out of my hair, it had felt like I had just conditioned it.

It should be noted though that, there is still a detox period using any natural method of no-pooing. If you have been using commercial shampoos in any capacity, your hair is going to need to both shed itself of all of the silicons and plasticizers as well as readjust its natural oil cycle. I did notice a MUCH shorter detox period from this recipe AND I found that it helped my color damaged cottage cheese hair repair faster thanks to the silica in the horsetail and oatstraw. I now only need to wash my hair once a week, after my hair finished detoxing.

INGREDEINTS

- 3 cups distilled water (I personally use a hydrosol to get the added benefits of herbs. My current mud cleanser in the shower, contains lime hydrosol)
- 2 Tbsp. marshmallow root (the slip that this provides really makes a difference in the end result. Though you can omit the "hair healing herbs" below, I would not omit the marshmallow root.)
- 4-6 Tbsp. hair healing herbs of choice (I personally ALWAYS make mine with 1 Tbsp. each of horsetail, oatstraw, nettle, green tea, and for an extra little bit of a red boost I add hibiscus. If given a choice of herbs for all hair types that really make this recipe awesome, I would say don't leave out the horsetail, oatstraw, and nettle. Horsetail and oatstraw contain high amounts of silica and this helps your hair feel much softer and grow much faster. Nettle contains a high amount of vitamins and minerals that are great for all hair types and helps to stimulate the scalp.)
- 1/2 cup apple cider vinegar
- 3/4 cup clay (You can use bentonite or rhassoul clay. I personally LOVE rhassoul clay and find that its high mineral content really makes a difference on my hair, but people with

oily hair/scalp might find bentonite clay helps to keep the oils at bay.)

- 1/4 cup aloe Vera gel
- 1 Tbsp. Carrier oil of choice
- essential oils of choice

DIRECTIONS

• This recipe is first a decoction. When using roots, especially mucilage giving roots like marshmallow root, it is better to release their healing properties by simmering the root in water (or hydrosol) for 15-20 minutes. Bring 3 cups water (or hydrosol) and marshmallow root to a boil and turn down to simmer for 15-20 minutes.

• After making the marshmallow root decoction, remove from heat and add hair healing herbs of your choice. Leave all of the herbs to steep until it's cool. Strain herbs, taking extra care to squeeze out the herbs to get all the extra tea.

• Combine 1 cup of herbal infusion/decoction with apple cider vinegar, clay, aloe Vera gel, and essential oils. Stir until completely mixed together. Store in an air tight container for a week in your bath tub (or longer if you add a few drops of a natural preservatives such as grapeseed extract, grapefruit seed extract, rosemary antioxidant, and/or colloidal silver. Refrigeration can also help keep your mud for several months.)

TO USE: Wet hair as you would when shampooing then pour some mud into your palm and begin cleansing your hair with it, starting from your roots and massaging down to the tips. Let sit for 5 minutes (don't let it dry) and then rinse clean. Follow with Silken Goddess apple cider vinegar rinse.

Dry Shampoo for Light or Dark Hair

Have you heard about dry shampoos yet? They seem to be all the rage among my friends, but I had never actually thought about using them myself. I am not sure why I hadn't tried dry shampoo yet, it's not like I take a shower every day...or even every other day. Shhhh....don't tell! You wouldn't know it because I smell like I have very peaceful pits (hehe), but making my hair look like it has been washed, when I clearly haven't had the time to wash it, sounds like a dream to me!

If you have never heard of them, dry shampoos are essentially a powder that you can apply to your dirty/greasy/unwashed hair to absorb and "clean" the excess oils from your scalp, making your hair look like it has just been washed. I was very excited to have a reason NOT to wash my hair, but then again who has the time to wash their hair every day? Not this busy hippy!

Many of the Popular Dry Shampoo Brands Contain Toxic Chemicals

I did my homework and started looking into the ingredients in the more popular brands (such ash Garnier Fructise, Aveeno, and Got 2b) that are sold at stores near you. It wasn't pretty. I found a large majority of them contain flammable chemicals such as propane and butane; not to mention fragrance, pthalates, and parabens! I wasn't dying to put butane and propane on my scalp, so I went on a search to see what I could make.

You Can Find Many Nourishing Ingredients Around Your Home

I didn't realize it at the time, but I already had ALL the ingredients I needed to make a fabulous dry shampoo. The basic recipe that floats around the web is cornstarch or arrowroot powder for light hair and cocoa powder combined with arrowroot powder for dark hair, but I wanted to make an exceptional dry shampoo that would help condition my hair and provide much needed nutrients too. After looking through my cabinets, I came up with a list of things that can be used in your dry shampoo recipe:

- ground oatmeal
- clays (white, french green, rhasoul, etc.)
- finely ground herbs (lavender, peppermint, rosemary, chamomile, calendula, roses, etc. These will add a nice light herbal scent to your dry shampoo and hair as well.)
- coconut milk powder
- baking soda (be careful using this. A friend of mine with sensitive skin used this as a dry shampoo and it made her skin get all red and peely!)
- cinnamon powder
- almond meal powder
- cornmeal and salt

I'd Choose Cinnamon Over Chocolate No Matter the

Reason

Whether it's for breakfast or which dark powder I am about to sprinkle upon my head, my first love is always sworn to cinnamon. It is exotic and delightful to the senses and has so many amazing antibacterial and healing properties, that I tend to favor it over other choices. Now don't get me wrong, in it's raw form, cacao is chock full of antioxidants, vitamins, and minerals, but I just can not help but add cinnamon to everything. My love for cinnamon runs really deep. If you do not have cocoa powder handy, cinnamon powder is a fabulous substitute, AND smells Ah-MAZE-ing.

My Hair Looked Like It Had Been Freshly Washed

With no knowledge of how awesome dry shampoos really can be, I was completely shocked to find that my hair turned out totally oil free and soft as can be. Not only that, it smelled absolutely delightful. I was most impressed by how clean my hair looked afterward. I had half expected to see remnants of the dry shampoo in my hair, but instead my hair looked clean.

DRY SHAMPOO FOR DARK HAIR INGREDEINTS

• 2 Tbsp. cocoa powder or cinnamon powder (I used organic fair trade raw cacao powder AND organic cinnamon bark powder. Both are chock full of nutrients that help to condition your hair.)
• 1 Tbsp. arrowroot powder (or non-gmo cornstarch)
• 1/2 Tbsp. coconut milk powder (optional, this can be replaced by arrowroot/cornstarch powder if you do not have this on hand. This will help condition your hair.)
• 1/2 Tbsp. finely ground oatmeal powder (optional, this can be replaced by arrowroot/cornstarch powder if you do now have this on hand.)
• 5-10 drops essential oil (optional. Lavender, rosemary, and peppermint essential oils are all great choices!)

DRY SHAMPOO FOR LIGHT HAIR INGREDEINTS

• 2 Tbsp. arrowroot powder (or non-gmo cornstarch)
• 1 Tbsp. coconut milk powder (optional, this can be replaced by arrowroot/cornstarch powder if you do not have this on hand. This will help condition your hair.)

- 1 Tbsp. finely ground oatmeal powder (optional, this can be replaced by arrowroot/cornstarch powder if you do now have this on hand.)
- 5-10 drops essential oil (optional. Lavender, rosemary, and peppermint essential oils are all great choices!)

DIRECTIONS

- Combine powdered ingredients until well blended. If adding essential oils, stir them in until combined.
- Using an old makeup blush brush, dust the dry shampoo onto the roots or oil parts of your hair. If you don't have an old makeup brush, you can just comb this dry shampoo through your hair.
- Store your homemade dry shampoo in a re-purposed container.

Natural Conditioners

While learning my way through natural hair care and the no-poo method, I have found that carrier oils by themselves, are very difficult to get out of your hair without shampoo and suds. This caused me to look in depth at other non-oil conditioner choices. There are actually many options out there, in you pantry alone, that you can use to condition your hair.

- Natural conditioners for hair
- Raw Unfiltered Honey – The great thing about honey is that it's water soluble, meaning it is easy to wash out of your hair without soapy bubbles. Not only does honey make a great no-poo alternative, but its extreme healing capabilities make it a wonderful deep conditioner too. Honey is a natural humectant (it helps to retain moisture) and emollient (it softens and smoothes). Honey's natural antibacterial and antioxidant properties have proven to help heal the scalp as well. (Note: honey also has a small amount of peroxide in it and can, over time, lighten your hair. Those with darker hair may want to use molasses instead, though a deep conditioning treatment every now and then has never shown any change in my hair color.) To use, you can either combine equal amounts with olive oil, over heat, or apply honey by itself. After applying roots to tip, cover your head with a shower cap and let sit for 10 minutes before no-pooing as usual.
- Molasses – Just like honey, molasses is water soluble and a natural humectant and emollient. Like it's lighter counterpart, molasses also has a ton of minerals and antioxidants. Molasses also contains a good

amount of B vitamins, which your hair happens to love! Use just like honey, but works best for darker hair rather than blonde.

• Oils – We all know that coconut oil, olive oil, hemp seed oil, etc. are fabulous treatments for our hair. Whenever I do a hot oil treatment in my hair, I always do it prior to my normal shampoo/no-poo routine. I have never been able to just simply rinse the oil out of my hair with solely water. My mud "shampoo" followed by a ACV rinse has worked for me in getting the coconut oil out of my hair after a deep conditioning treatment.

• Henna/Senna/Indigo – This is one of my favorite deep conditioners to use on my hair! Henna, a green grassy smelling plant powder used to dye hair and skin, also naturally strengthens and conditions your hair by penetrating the shaft of the hair and filling in gaps. True henna colors the hair lightly with red undertones. For blonde hair it's best to use Senna or neutral "henna" (also known as cassia), it does all the conditioning but none of the red color. For black hair indigo is used. More on henna and natural hair coloring in the next post!

• Aloe Vera – With a pH of around 4.5, aloe very makes a wonderful conditioner for our hair because it naturally helps to close the cuticle. Aloe Vera also helps to soften hair, as well as to heal dandruff and other scalp conditions. It also helps with hair loss and hair growth!

• Avocado – Avocados are extremely good for hair! They are chock full of vitamins B and E, making them great to help with hair loss and hair growth. Their high fat content actually helps to deeply penetrate the shaft of the hair, conditioning your hair from the inside out. You can either just mash that avocado and apply directly to your hair, or add a Tbsp. of carrier oil for an extra deep conditioner.

• Bananas - I was going to talk about how awesome bananas are because of all the vitamins and minerals they contain that your hair loves…but in the making of this post I made a banana hair mask and must have not combed my hair properly beforehand or something because it took me 20 minutes to get the banana out of my hair. It caused my hair to tangle so badly that I ended up losing a good deal of hair just trying to get it out…I would suggest you combine banana with a carrier oil and blend VERY well in a blender/food processor, if you are going to put it in your hair for a conditioner. The oil combined with it blended well enough that there are no chunks, should help keep it from making your hair a sticky mess if you choose to use this option.

• Coconut Milk - Just like coconut oil, coconut milk can benefit your hair in many ways. It is often used in hair masks and fills up your hair with proteins. Rich in vitamins, minerals, and fatty acids, coconut milk can help with hair loss/growth, luster, softness, and SOOO much more. You can make a great 2-in-1 no-poo/conditioner with aloe Vera and coconut milk!

• Eggs – Eggs are an excellent choice for a natural deep conditioner. Not only does the yolk, rich in fats and proteins, naturally moisturize your hair, but the whites, containing bacteria-eating enzymes, help to remove excess oils from your hair and scalp. I love to use eggs in my deep conditioning henna hair mix but you can just whip 2 raw eggs and apply to your hair alone if you don't have all of the other herbal ingredients.

Marshmallow Root Herbal Detangling Spray

I LOVE this spray! With no oils in it, this spray always leaves my hair soft but not oily at all. The marshmallow root is essential to this spray, giving it the "slip" that aids in detangling your hair. This spray is absolutely wonderful to use on small children who hate to have their hair combed! Add in some calming essential oils such as lavender and chamomile (which also have great healing effects for the hair too) and use this on your child's hair right before bed! I have also used this spray as a pre-wash before using my mud shampoo. I use it to detangle my hair before washing with the mud, to make it easier!

INGREDEINTS

- 3 cups distilled water
- 2 Tbsp. marshmallow root (this is the herb that gives this spray it's slip for ultra awesome detangling power!)
- 4-6 Tbsp. hair healing herbs of choice (I personally ALWAYS make mine with 1 Tbsp. each of horsetail, oatstraw, nettle, green tea, and for an extra little bit of a red boost I add hibiscus, but you could add chamomile for blonde hair or rosemary for dark hair. If given a choice of herbs for all hair types that really make this recipe awesome, I would say don't leave out the horsetail, oatstraw, and nettle.)
- 1/4 cup aloe Vera gel
- 1/2 cup distilled water/hydrosol (This is for the actual spray itself.)
- 20 drops essential oils of choice
- 8 oz. spray bottle

DIRECTIONS

•   (This decoction/herbal infusion is also the same one I use for my herbal mud shampoo) This recipe is first a decoction. When using roots, especially mucilage giving roots like marshmallow root, it is better to release their healing properties by simmering the root in water (or hydrosol) for 15-20 minutes. Bring 3 cups water (or hydrosol) and marshmallow root to a boil and turn down to simmer for 15-20 minutes.

•   After making the marshmallow root decoction, remove from heat and add hair healing herbs of your choice. Leave all of the herbs to steep until it's cool. Strain herbs, taking extra care to squeeze out the herbs to get all the extra tea.

•   Combine 1/4 cup of the marshmallow root decoction/herbal infusion with 1/4 cup aloe Vera gel, essential oils, and water/hydrosol to fill the spray bottle. Keep in the fridge to keep longer. You can also add a few drops of colloidal silver or grapeseed extract/grapefruit seed extract for longer preservation.

TO USE: Always SHAKE the bottle before use. Spray generously on wet (or dry) hair and brush or comb through hair.

Heavenly Hippy Hair – Deep Conditioning Hair Mask

This hair mask doesn't smell the greatest but it makes my hair so soft and ultra conditioned while adding depth and color, that I am willing to withstand the smell of grassy apple cider vinegar while I am making it. It is WELL worth it in the end! I usually use this hair mask once every two weeks, but it can be used once a week if you need it that badly. If you are trying to go no-poo, this hair mask will greatly accelerate you through the detox period. People with extremely damaged and color treated hair have a difficult time during the detox process of no-pooing, and this helps to fill in the holes in your hair caused by all of that damage; making the transition easier on your hair. Whenever my hair got overly oily and dull, during the detox period, I just whipped up this mask and came out with lovely hair once again.

HEAVENLY HIPPY HAIR – DRY MIX

INGREDIENTS

•   2 parts henna (this doesn't have to be colored henna, you can get the neutral henna, also known as cassia or senna, for just the conditioning properties of the herb itself, though henna is not like chemical color treatments. It is much more natural looking and will not come out with roots as your hair is growing. It only enhances the beauty of your hair rather than drastically changing it's color like conventional dyes.)

- 2 parts horsetail, finely ground
- 1 part oatstraw, finely ground
- 1 part nettle, finely ground
- 1 part color enhancing herb, finely ground (I use hibiscus or calendula for red hair, chamomile or lemon peel for blonde hair, and sage or rosemary for dark hair)
- **HAIR MASK INGREDIENTS**

- 3/4 cup apple cider vinegar (Coconut milk, hydrosol, or water can be replaced here if needed, but the ACV helps to further condition hair and some even say it helps your hair to absorb more of the color from the henna)
- 2 beaten eggs
- 1/4 cup aloe Vera gel
- 2 Tbsp. oil of your choice (You can use coconut oil, olive oil, hemp seed oil, etc. This oil can also be optional, but is very hydrating and washes out just fine with the herbal ingredients. I have never had my hair left oily from adding it into my hair mask)
- 1/2 cup Heavenly Hippy Hair Mix
- 20 drops essential oil (optional - chamomile and lavender are both very healing to the hair and scalp. Rosemary and basil can help with hair growth, and carrot seed is fabulous for dry brittle hair)

DIRECTIONS

•   Combine all of the powdered ingredients for the Heavenly Hippy Hair Dry Mix, in a glass bowl (not metal, metal reacts with henna in the same manner that it does with conventional hair dyes.) Store powdered mix in a mason jar with a plastic lid or a plastic container. Will keep for a year or two, as long as no moisture is introduced.

•   In a small pan, combine apple cider vinegar (or water/hydrosol) and 1/2 cup of Heavenly Hippy Hair Mix. Stir over medium heat for 5 minutes. Don't let it boil!

•   Let mixture cool for 5 minutes and then mix in beaten eggs, oil, and essential oils.

- Apply to hair working from root to tips. Wrap head in plastic wrap or cover with a shower cap and then wrap with a warm damp towel around your head. You are trying to keep as much heat in as possible!
- Leave on hair for a minimum of 45 minutes up to 2 hours depending on the amount of color you want in your hair. It will never be so bold as chemical hair dye treatments, so leaving it on even for 2 hours still will look natural and beautiful.
- Rinse from hair with warm/cool water in the shower. It may take a few minutes to fully get the herbs out of your hair. There is no need to shampoo (or no-poo) your hair after this. Pretend this was your no-poo and follow with a diluted apple cider vinegar rinse (I use a 32 oz spray bottle and combine 1/4 cup ACV, 1/4 cup aloe Vera gel, water to fill, and essential oils. I spray my hair until it's soaked with the ACV rinse and then comb my hair through. You can either rinse clean or leave in to dry in your hair. It won't smell of ACV when your hair dries.)

Natural Herbal Hair Color for Healthy Hair

I have spent a lot of years of my life changing my hair color based on my flittering emotions and the change of seasons. I am a big proponent of self expression and coloring my hair has always been one of my favorite ways to express myself, but over the last few years I have come to find out that all of those conventional hair dyes I was using is absolutely terrible for me and for the planet.

Over time, I was destroying my hair and ingesting nasty toxic chemicals, with every dye job that I performed. Finally after wanting to grow my hair out, I realized that my hair had never gotten passed my shoulders because all of the damage I was doing to it was causing my hair to break off. I decided I needed to make a change and how I was coloring my hair was the first thing on that list.

After trying henna, I don't think I can ever go back to conventional hair dyes. I mean, the toxic chemicals is enough on its own to keep me away for good...but the conditioning that henna provides to your hair is simply divine, all while coloring it. I can not profess enough my love for henna.

Conventional hair dyes contain dangerous ingredients

Not only does conventional hair dye destroy your hair by turning it into Swiss cheese, but the use of conventional hair dye has been linked to cancer, allergic reactions, and respiratory disorders. hair dyes that are marked as "natural" can be deceiving too, because they can contain hazardous chemicals such as resorcinol, ammonia or peroxide, and PPD. PPD is widely known to damage the DNA of human cells and often causes allergic reactions in even mildly sensitive individuals. Studies have shown that those who use conventional hair dyes are at an increased risk of developing Hodgkin's lymphoma, multiple myeloma, and leukemia. My sister-in-law once had such a bad reaction to dyeing her hair that she had to go to the emergency room because her whole face had swollen up like she had just been in a boxing match!

Henna makes my heart swell

My favorite way to color my hair is with henna. I REALLY love using henna because not only are you coloring your hair, but you are also getting a nice deep conditioning too! Henna is a shrub that is native to the Middle East, West Asia, and North Africa. After harvest, the leaves are dried and pulverized into a fine powder. Henna has been used since ancient times to dye hair, skin, and nails. There's even been mention of Cleopatra using henna on her hair.

Henna penetrates the hair shaft and binds with the keratin in the hair making your hair stronger. Henna also coats the hair and fills in rough spots on frayed cuticles, adding a second layer of strength without locking out moisture.

Herbs for natural hair color

There are quite a few herbs, vegetable/fruits, and spices that you can use to color your hair. Most of these herbs and spices also have wonderful healing properties for your hair and scalp too. Herbs like rosemary are great for scalp conditions and hair growth. Herbs in bold are my favorite choices to use for that hair color.

Blonde Hair - Chamomile, Calendula, Lemon peel, Sunflower petals, Saffron (golden highlights that you can use on brown as well) Marigold, Catnip, Mullein flowers, Honey

Red Hair - Calendula, Marigold, Henna, Hibiscus flowers, Red Clover flowers, Rose hips, Red Rose petals, Beets, Carrots, Rooibos tea

Brown Hair - Black Walnut Hulls, Black Tea, Nettle, Rosemary, Sage, Comfrey root, Coffee, Cherry tree bark, Cloves, Cinnamon,

Black Hair - Black Walnut Hulls, Black Tea, Coffee, Indigo

Helping your hair color stay longer

By prepping your hair before and after hair coloring you can get the most color in your hair and make it last longer. If you use a mordant prior to coloring and a final rinse with a fixative, you can help your hair hold the color longer.

Herbal Mordants - Plants high in tannins used before coloring can help open up the hair shaft to accept more color during the color process. Simply make a strong infusion with one of the two and rinse hair. Leave in for 30 minutes, rinse, and towel dry. Move on to the color phase.

black tea – great for darker colors

catnip – great for lighter colors

Natural Color Fixatives - When used after hair coloring, fixatives helps the color to last longer. Most fixatives can be drying to your hair but Apple Cider Vinegar, used as a hair rinse, is the perfect natural option that helps to close the cuticles as well as softens the hair. Simply combine 1 Tbsp. ACV with 8 oz. of water (I like to also add 1 Tbsp. aloe Vera gel as well) in a spray bottle and spray onto hair after coloring hair. Don't rinse out.

Herbal Hair Coloring "Mud"

DRY MIX INGREDIENTS

•   3 parts henna, cassia, or indigo (depending on the color you are trying to achieve henna for red and browns, indigo for browns and blacks, and cassia for blondes. To make it easiest you can simply pick out which hair color you are looking for at Mountain Rose Herbs! They have the best hair coloring henna I have tried; not all hennas are created equal.)
•   1 part finely ground hair coloring herbs (see above for herbs to use. Combining herbs can create varying desired shades)

MUD INGREDIENTS

•   1/2 cup dry coloring mix
•   3/4 cup apple cider vinegar (Coconut milk, hydrosol, or water can be replaced here if needed, but the ACV helps to further condition hair and also helps your hair to absorb more of the color from the henna)

- 1 Tbsp. carrier oil (optional – for dry hair, you can use coconut, almond, hemp, olive, etc.)

DIRECTIONS

- Combine all of the powdered ingredients for the Dry Mix, in a glass bowl (not metal, metal reacts with henna in the same manner that it does with conventional hair dyes.) Store powdered mix in a mason jar with a plastic lid or a plastic container. Will keep for a year or two, as long as no moisture is introduced.
- In a small pan, combine apple cider vinegar (or coconut milk/water/hydrosol) and 1/2 cup of dry mix. Stir over medium heat for 5 minutes. Don't let it boil!
- Let mixture cool for 5 minutes and then mix in carrier oil.
- Henna may be applied to wet or dry hair that is clean. Apply a cream or oil around your hairline, ears, and neck to avoid staining your skin. This applies to your hands, so wear gloves! Apply to hair working from root to tips. Wrap head in plastic wrap or cover with a shower cap and then wrap with a warm damp towel around your head. You are trying to keep as much heat in as possible!
- Leave on hair for a minimum of 45 minutes up to 2 hours depending on the amount of color you want impart into your hair. It will never be so bold as chemical hair dye treatments, so leaving it on even for 2 hours still will look natural and beautiful.
- Rinse from hair with warm/cool water in the shower. It may take a few minutes to fully get the herbs out of your hair. There is no need to shampoo (or no-poo) your hair after this. If you have herbs stuck in your hair, it is easiest to let your hair dry then they will easily fall out of your hair. Follow with Silken Goddess apple cider vinegar rinse.

Herbal Color Tea Rinse

This herbal color tea will impart a very light natural color into your hair. It has a stacking effect though, so frequent use can help you to attain the darker shades that you may be desiring. For both light and dark hair, you can achieve slightly more dramatic results by sitting for the 1 hour out in the sun. Heat is what you are trying to attain, so a blow dryer can be used in place of the sun, but to conserve energy I suggest spraying your hair until wet with color tea, blow drying until dry, and then repeating several times before rinsing, rather than drying your hair for an entire hour...who wants to hold the dryer up that long anyway?

INGREDEINTS

- 1/2 cup hair coloring herbs (see above)
- 2 cups boiling hot distilled water
- 1/4 cup aloe Vera gel - optional, I love to add this for the extra healing boost it gives to my hair as well as for its capabilities of balancing your hair's pH.
- 1 Tbsp. honey/molasses - optional, both are conditioning to the hair. Use honey for light hair and molasses for dark hair.

DIRECTIONS

•   Steep herbs in water for 1+ hours. Some herbs that provide lighter hair colors, such as chamomile, benefit from boiling for 30 minutes rather than steeping in boiling water. I like to steep until the water is cool enough to use. Strain herbs using tea strainer/cheese cloth/etc., making sure to squeeze out all the extra juice from the herbs.

•   Combine with aloe Vera gel and honey/molasses, if using, and put into a spray bottle. You can use this rinse by just pouring it over your hair from a bowl, but I find using a spray bottle helps to control the mess and waste. If using a bowl, I suggest using a second bowl to hold your head over so that you can reuse the tea over your hair several times.

•   Leave on your hair for one hour, then rinse the tea out and follow with apple cider vinegar rinse. For even more "dramatic" results, spend the hour out in the sun.

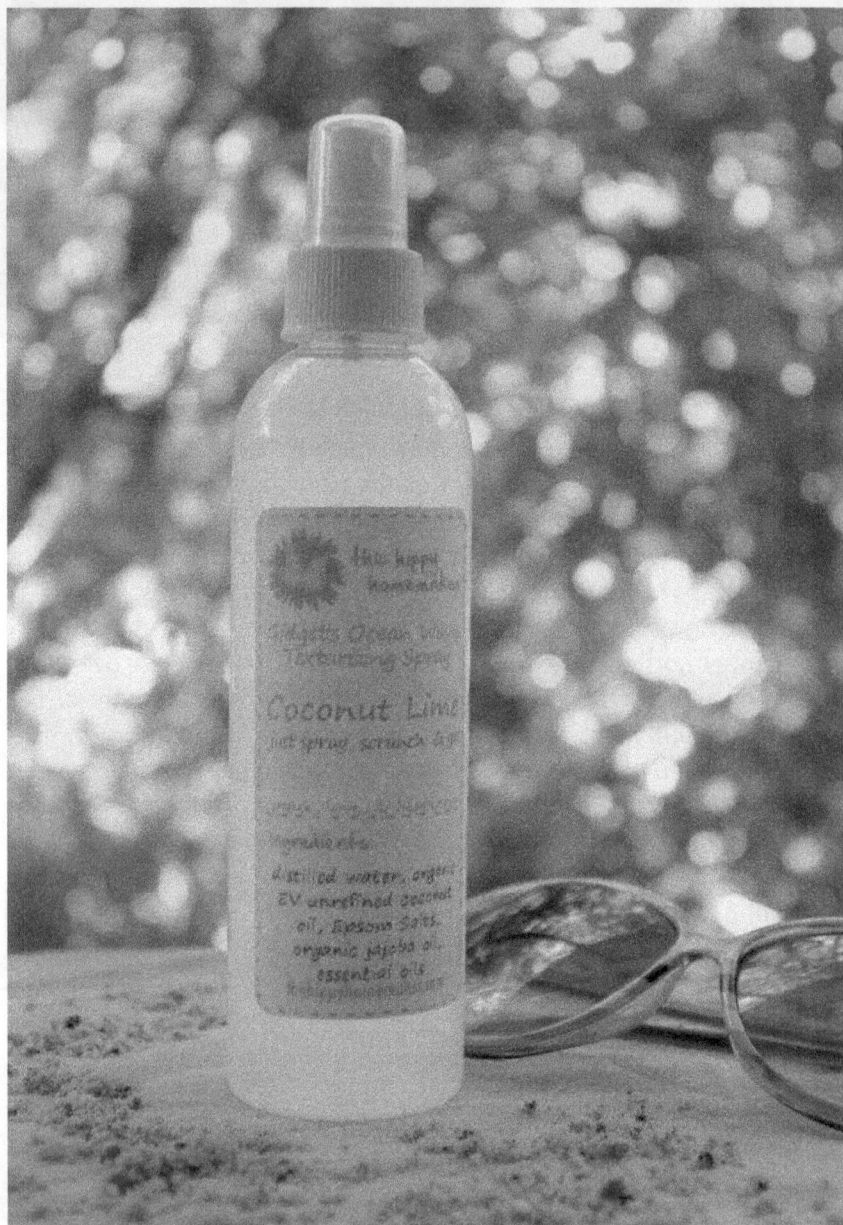

Gidget's Ocean Waves Sea Salt Texturizing Hair Spray

Everyone loves the tousled, messed up waves that you get when you go to the beach, but not everyone has a beach at their back door. This is why I created Gidget's (my nickname!) Ocean Waves Texturizing Spray. Not only does this awesome spray condition and texturize your hair, it also smells great without all of the harmful chemicals in it!

You can make this spray in three different holds, without the sugar if all you want is a sea salt texturizing spray, regular hold which is made with a small amount of sugar for just a natural hold, or heavy hold with extra sugar for those who don't have naturally curly or wavy hair.

INGREDEINTS

- 1 Tbsp. Epsom salt
- ½ Tbsp. Sea salt (I use dead sea salt and pink Himalayan salt here)
- 1 Tbsp. Aloe Vera gel
- ½ tsp. Conditioner (I like to use the Dr. Bronner's leave in conditioner for this)
- 1 Tbsp. Vegetable glycerin (*optional* – this helps add moisture and controls frizz)
- **Regular Hold** – 1 Tbsp. Sugar
- **Heavy Hold** – 2 Tbsp. Sugar
- water to fill
- 8 oz. Spray bottle
- essential oils (My favorite options for this spray is 10 drops each of lavender and grapefruit, but I do also really love the rosemary lime version as well and rosemary is great for helping your hair grow by stimulating the scalp.)

DIRECTIONS

• Heat 1 cup of water to boiling and remove from heat. Stir in all other ingredients until dissolved. Pour into 8 oz. Spray bottle.

TO USE: Always SHAKE the bottle before use. Spray generously on wet (or dry) hair and scrunch hair, then let air dry. Instead of air drying, you can also dry with a diffusor on your blow dryer, to get more volume and tighter waves/curls (depending on your hair type of course).

Easy Homemade Hair Spray

You would not believe just how simple it is to make a really effective hairspray that is not terrible for the environment! It only takes 3 ingredients to make this too! To change the hold of your hairspray, all you have to do is adjust the sugar levels. For a heavier hold add more sugar to the recipe. For a lighter hold, use less sugar in the recipe.

INGREDEINTS

- 1 ½ cups distilled water
- 2 Tbsp. white sugar
- 1 Tbsp. High proof alcohol (vodka is the best choice here and usually the cheapest)

DIRECTIONS

• Boil water and dissolve sugar in it. Allow to cool to room temp and then add alcohol.

• Store in a spray bottle and use as your regular hairspray.

NOTE: For a stronger hold you can adjust the sugar up, and for less stiffness adjust the sugar down.

Head Trip Hair Pomade

My husband is a drummer in a rock band and when he has his 'hawk growing, he is in need of a good beeswax pomade to help hold his hair up. I designed this hair pomade to help strengthen and condition your hair while holding the 'do in place and/or texturizing your style. The addition of organic unrefined Shea butter and organic jojoba oil, you will be conditioning your hair while you use it! There are two different holds with this recipe. The medium hold is a softer hold that works well with texturizing hair rather than holding something in place. For the bed head look or soft smooth curls, the medium hold is perfect! The Heavy hold is the hold that the Hippy Hubby likes to use for his 'hawk. Most of my male clients tend to purchase the heavy hold more often. You can even style a pompadour with the heavy hold!

MEDIUM HOLD INGREDEINTS

- 3 Tbsp. Unrefined Shea butter
- 2 Tbsp. Beeswax pastilles
- 2 Tbsp. Jojoba oil (You can substitute other carrier oils here but jojoba oil is by far the best oil for hair care since it is the same composition as our skin's sebum.)

HEAVY HOLD INGREDEINTS

- 3 Tbsp. Beeswax pastilles
- 2 Tbsp. Unrefined Shea butter

- 2 Tbsp. Jojoba oil (You can substitute other carrier oils here but jojoba oil is by far the best oil for hair care since it is the same composition as our skin's sebum.)

DIRECTIONS

- In a double boiler, combine ingredients and melt. Once melted, allow to sit on the heat for 20 minutes to process the Shea butter. Remove from heat.
- Pour oil/butter/wax mixture into a medium bowl. If adding essential oils and vitamin e to this recipe, pour in now.
- Using your hand mixer, blend the liquid as it starts to cool. Once it is the consistency of pudding, you can scoop into tins to further cool and harden. Store in a cool dark place when not in use.

TO USE: Dab a small penny sized amount of pomade onto your fingers and rub between fingers until spread evenly. Apply to hair until desired amount has been used and style achieved.

Flax Seed Hair Gel

Flax seeds are filled with omega-3's and essential fatty acids that are great for hair growth, hair softness, and hair luster and shine. This flax seed hair gel is really fantastic for curly haired girls! It lends the perfect amount of hold without any of the crunchiness, leaving your hair silky soft.

INGREDEINTS

- ¼ cup whole brown flax seeds
- 2 cups distilled water (hydrosol or aloe Vera juice can be substituted here)

DIRECTIONS

- Simmer for 8-10 minutes until gel is starting to thicken. You don't want to overcook the gel, as this will make it too thick to strain out. It will thicken further as it cools.
- Strain through a fine metal strainer, and store in the fridge for up to two weeks.

TO USE: Scoop out a small mount and work into hair, styling as usual. For beautiful soft curls, I apply to my hair while it's wet. I scrunch and dry my hair with a diffusor on my blow dryer to create the most bouncy soft curls.

Vegan Agar Agar Seaweed Hair Gel

For a heavier hold vegan hair gel, flax isn't always the right answer. This is where nourishing seaweed comes into play! Seaweed is known to be extremely rich in vitamins and minerals that help promote hair growth. Rich in antioxidants and omega-3's, seaweed is known to contain up to twenty times the elements of land plants.

INGREDEINTS

- 1 tsp. Agar agar flakes (you can use up to 1 more tsp. of agar agar powder to make a heavier hold)
- 1 cup water (you can substitute hydrosol or coconut milk here)
- ¼ cup aloe Vera gel
- 5 drops rosemary essential oil (*optional)*
- 5 drops lime peel essential oil (*optional*)
- 3 drops vanilla absolute (*optional*)

DIRECTIONS

•   In a small pan, heat the water to a boil. Turn the heat down to simmer and slowly whisk in the agar agar powder.

•   Whisk until the agar agar is completely dissolved. If it is not, it will leave clumps in the gel. Once completely dissolved, remove from heat and add aloe Vera gel.

•   Store in sealed jar in the fridge, when not in use.

TO USE: Scoop a small amount out of the jar and style your hair accordingly.

Gelatin Hair Gel

If you are more likely to have some really good grass fed gelatin in your pantry, instead of the agar agar powder, you can make a hair gel that is just as awesome! Gelatin is high in collagen helping to strengthen your hair and promote hair growth.

INGREDEINTS

•   **Light Hold -** ½ tsp. gelatin

- **Medium Hold –** ¾ tsp. gelatin
- **Heavy Hold –** 1 tsp. gelatin

- 1 cup distilled water
- ¼ cup aloe Vera gel (*optional* – this helps to keep your hair from drying out, but is not needed to make this recipe work)

DIRECTIONS

•   Heat water enough to dissolve gelatin. Whisk gelatin in until it's completely dissolved.

•   Pour gelatin into a bowl and put in the fridge for a couple hours, to set up.

•   Once completely cool, scoop into a blender or food processor and add the aloe Vera gel. Blend until mixed together.

•   Store in a jar in the fridge for two weeks.

TO USE: Scoop a small amount out of the jar and style your hair accordingly.

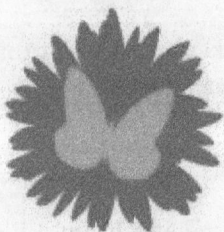

Chapter 9

Hand & Foot Care

Our hands and feet tend to get the roughest treatment from us. Every day we use them for pretty much every task we have at hand. Calluses, blisters, funky smelling feet, and cleaning dirty hands that have been in the garden, can easily be taken care of in the comfort of your own home.

Soothing Peppermint Lavender Foot Scrub

This soothing tingly foot scrub will scour away any dead skin cells, revive tired feet, and leave your skin soft as a baby's butt. You can choose to do a lavender lemon option for a fresh summertime scent, just replace the peppermint essential oil with lemon essential oil.

INGREDIENTS

- 1 cup sea salt
- ¼ cup baking soda
- ½ cup coconut oil
- 10 drops peppermint essential oil
- 15 drops lavender essential oil

DIRECTIONS

• Combine ingredients in a bowl. Store in a jar in a cool dark place, when not in use.

TO USE: Soak feet in warm/hot water for 10 minutes. It's even better if you use the Soothing Herbal Foot Soak rather than just water. With clean dry hands, scoop out a Tablespoon or so and scrub feet well, making sure to get rougher areas really well. Rinse with warm water and pat feet dry with a towel. Follow with hand/foot butter and cover with socks to lock in moisture over night.

Soothing Herbal Foot Soak

This herbal foot soak is designed to soothe achy muscles, relax tired feet, and to soften leathery skin. You can substitute the herbs in this recipe for other herbs that you might have on hand or in your garden. This can be followed with a foot scrub or pumice on softened calluses. This is recommended for athletes or people who spend all day on their feet. The essential oils can be omitted from this recipe if you do not have them on hand.

- Foot tub
- ½ cup Epsom salts
- 2 Tbsp. Raw apple cider vinegar
- 2 Tbsp. dried or ¼ cup fresh rosemary
- 2 Tbsp. dried or ¼ cup fresh basil
- 2 Tbsp. chamomile flowers
- 2 Tbsp. Lavender buds
- 10 drops lavender essential oil
- 5 drops roman chamomile essential oil
- 3 drops clove essential oil
- 3 drops sweet marjoram essential oil

DIRECTIONS

• Combine Epsom salt, essential oils, and herbs in a glass bowl. Mix until combined evenly.

TO USE: Pour Soothing Herbal Bath mixture into foot tub filled with warm/hot water. Mix up until salts are dissolved and stick your feet in to soak for 15 to 20 minutes. Gently pat feet dry and follow with hand/foot butter.

Foot Deodorizing Powder

This foot powder is designed with herbs that have astringent properties and are known to be great deodorizers to help freshen sweaty odorous feet.

INGREDEINTS

- ¼ cup white kaolin clay

135

- ¼ cup arrowroot powder
- 2 Tbsp. Baking soda
- 1 Tbsp. Finely ground sage
- 1 Tbsp. Finely ground lavender buds
- 1 Tbsp. Finely ground rosemary
- 10 drops lavender essential oil
- 5 tea tree essential oil
- 10 drops lemon essential oil
- 2 drops geranium essential oil

DIRECTIONS

•   Combine powdered ingredients in a bowl. Mix in essential oils. I find it easiest to evenly mix essential oils into powders such as this, by using my fingers to mix the powder.

TO USE: Sprinkle powder into dry shoes to deodorize shoes and keep them smelling fresh and stink-free.

Fungus Amungus Anti-Fungal Foot Powder

This is a very effective anti-fungal foot powder. If used often, on clean dry feet, this foot powder can help with athlete's foot and more!

INGREDEINTS

- ¼ cup arrowroot powder
- ¼ cup white kaolin clay
- 1 Tbsp. Finely ground chaparral
- 1 Tbsp. Finely ground black walnut hulls
- 1 Tbsp. Finely ground lavender buds
- 25 drops lavender essential oil
- 20 drops tea tree essential oil
- 10 drops clove essential oil
- 10 drops red thyme essential oil

DIRECTIONS

•   Combine powdered ingredients in a bowl. Mix in essential oils. I find it easiest to evenly mix essential oils into powders such as this, by using my fingers to mix the powder.

TO USE: Sprinkle powder into dry shoes and onto clean dry feet daily, to keep feet fungal free and to keep athlete's foot at bay.

Citrus Revitalizing Hand Scrub

The very first time that I used a hand scrub was in a store that shall be left nameless. I was completely shocked at how incredibly soft and smooth my hands felt after receiving this exfoliating scrub. From then on out, I was obsessed with exfoliation and have created a plethora of different exfoliating scrub ideas. This Citrus Revitalizing Hand Scrub is awesome because it serves multiple functions rather than just exfoliation. The citrus in this scrub is great at whitening dull nails and giving your skin a drink in vitamin C magic, while the sugar and oil help to lock in moisture.

INGREDEINTS

- 1 cup sugar
- ¼ cup lemon peel powder (or lemon and lime zest)
- ¼ cup coconut oil
- 2 Tbsp. olive oil
- 10 drops lemon essential oil
- 15 drops sweet orange essential oil

DIRECTIONS

• Combine ingredients in a bowl. Store in a jar in a cool dark place, when not in use.

TO USE: With clean dry hands, scoop out a Tablespoon or so and scrub hands in a gentle circular motion. Rinse with warm water and pat hands dry with a towel. Follow with hand/foot butter and cover with gloves to lock in moisture over night.

Healing Nail & Cuticle Butter

This butter is very easy to make and is super nourishing to the cuticles and nails. Use this while doing your nails and trimming your cuticles. Dab a small amount onto each of your cuticles and massage into them before pushing them down and trimming them.

INGREDEINTS

- ¼ cup unrefined coconut oil
- ¼ cup extra virgin olive oil

- ¼ cup Shea butter
- ¼ cup beeswax pastilles
- ½ tsp. Lavender essential oil
- ½ tsp. Vitamin e
- 30 drops lemon essential oil
- 20 drops geranium essential oil

DIRECTIONS

•   Combine coconut oil, olive oil, Shea butter, and beeswax in a double boiler. Once melted, let sit on the heat for 20 minutes to process the Shea butter.

•   Remove from heat and add vitamin e and essential oils. Pour into tins or a mason jar and keep in a cool dark location when not in use.

TO USE: Dab a small amount onto each cuticle. Massage butter into cuticles and nails before pushing cuticles down and trimming them.

Nourishing Nail & Cuticle Oil

Blah blah blah

INGREDEINTS

- 2 Tbsp. Extra virgin olive oil (this is even better if you infuse the olive oil in calendula or use the Magic Healing oil from Chapter 10)
- 1 Tbsp. Unrefined coconut oil
- 1 tsp. Vitamin e
- 5 drops lavender essential oil
- 3 drops lemon essential oil
- 2 drops geranium essential oil

DIRECTIONS

•   Combine ingredients in a glass bottle with a dropper. Store in a cool dark location when not in use.

TO USE: Drop one single drop on each nail bed and massage into cuticles and nails.

Grapefruit Lavender Foaming Hand Soap

I find myself with a dilemma every single time that we go out to dinner to a restaurant. I bring Syfy with me to the bathroom to go potty (at this stage in my life, that's what it's called), and when we're finished, the usual hand washing routine comes upon us. I dread this when we're out, because the soap that is in nearly every bathroom, contains ingredients that I don't want to use on our skin. I used to have to debate it in my head, the lesser of two evils, until one day I bought a small 4 oz. Foaming soap dispenser. Absolutely the best $2 of my life. With this awesome little bottle that I keep in my purse, I can whip out the soap for Syfy and me, any time we need it and I feel great about what we are putting on our skin.

INGREDEINTS

- 4 oz. Foaming soap dispenser
- 1 tsp. Liquid castile soap
- 1 tsp. Carrier oil (hemp seed, olive oil, almond oil, etc.)
- water to fill
- 10 drops lavender essential oil
- 10 drops grapefruit essential oil
- 5 drops lemon essential oil

DIRECTIONS

• Combine ingredients, the soap last to prevent foaming over. Pump foaming soap out of container whenever needed.

Mechanic Hands – Hand Cleaner

Let me tell you...I used to be a sales manager at a car shop and the dirty hands that mechanics have cannot be rivaled by any other profession. The black grease and grime gets stuck in every crevice of the fingernails leaving them always dirty, even after a thorough hand washing. The top orange based hand soaps that we used in the shop, were actually toxic chemical laden detergents masquerading as a soap. I first made this recipe as a soft scrub for my sinks, bathtubs, and toilets, but it turns out that this recipe makes one of the most awesome mechanic hands cleansing soap.

My dad loves to ride his motorcycles, but owning a motorcycle isn't all riding. My dad spends a great deal of time personally taking care of his baby and that care usually leads to dirty mechanic hands. This hand scrub is his go-to scrub to get his hands grime-free after hours of working in the garage on his baby (the motorcycle).

INGREDEINTS

- 3 cups baking soda
- ½ cup liquid castile soap
- ½ cup water
- 40 drops sweet orange oil
- 25 drops lavender essential oil
- 20 drops lemon essential oil

DIRECTIONS

•   Combine ingredients in a bowl and mix thoroughly. Store in a jar with a lid. If it is too dry after storage, just add a small amount of water to mix into it again.

TO USE: Scoop a small amount onto hands with a spoon (so as to keep your dirt out of the clean soap) and scrub hands for several minutes with soap. Repeat if necessary. Follow with hand/foot butter.

Magic Hands Ultra Healing Hand & Foot Butter

This butter is really great at putting the moisture back into your hands and feet. Use this after exfoliating hands or feet, right before bed, or right after herbal soaks. If you slather this onto rough hands and feet, cover with socks or gloves, and leave overnight, you will find the most amazing results in the morning.

INGREDEINTS

- ¼ cup Shea butter
- ¼ cup cocoa butter
- ¼ cup coconut oil
- ¼ cup olive oil (Make this butter even more healing by substituting the Magic Healing Infused Oil from Chapter 10)
- 1 Tbsp. Arrowroot powder
- 1 Tbsp. Vitamin e
- 50 drops lavender essential oil
- 15 drops roman chamomile essential oil
- 15 drops geranium essential oil
- 3 drops carrot seed essential oil
- 10 drops frankincense essential oil

DIRECTIONS

• Combine butters and coconut oil in a double boiler to melt. Once melted, let sit on the heat for 20 minutes to process the butters. Remove from heat.

• In a small bowl, whisk together the olive oil, arrowroot powder, and vitamin e. Pour the liquid oil mixture and essential oils to the melted butter mixture. Stir until combined and pour into tin containers. Let sit to cool and harden. This recipe can be whipped in the same manner as the whipped body butter recipe in Chapter 4.

TO USE: Apply a medium thick layer onto hands or feet and cover with socks or gloves. Leave on overnight to heal and moisturize like magic! In the morning your hands and feet will be extremely soft. This is also great for aging skin and wrinkles! It makes my hands look ten years younger every time that I use it!

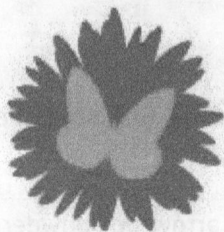

Chapter 10

The Magic of Herbal Infusions in Natural Health & Beauty

The great thing about DIY natural health and beauty recipes, is trying to find ways to incorporate more healing herbs into your recipes. There are so many different ways to infuse a recipe with herbs, you just have to get creative! You can infuse the different healing properties of herbs into oils, butters, apple cider vinegar, witch hazel, water, vegetable glycerin, and alcohol. Any of the recipes in this book can be easily upgraded with an herbal boost through infusion.

It is best, if possible, to avoid infusing water in the recipe, unless you are using the product right away. Water infusions last only a few days, up to a week, in the fridge before turning rancid and getting moldy.

Herbal Infused Oils

Making an herbal infused oil is extremely simple. All that you need is an organic healing carrier oil (olive, coconut, almond, grapeseed, hemp, etc.), the herbs of your choice, a mason jar, and some heat via the oven, sunshine, double boiler, etc. as long as it's very low heat (100-140 degrees F) so that you don't destroy the healing properties within the oil. When you steep the chosen herbs into your oil, you will be transferring those medicinal benefits from the plant into the oil. You can then use that oil in your healing recipes such as salves, massage oils, and even body butters. There are several methods that you can utilize to extract the herbal healing benefits into your oil.

Solar Infusion Method

This is one of the best methods to extract the healing benefits that your chosen herbs have. Not only are you charging your oil with naturally healing sun rays but this is the gentlest method of infusion. Some people also like to steep their herbs in moonlight, this can give it an extra boost as well. To infuse your oil solar style, just fill your jar 1/4-1/2 full of your herbs. You can do a single herb or even a combination depending on what you are planning to use your oil for. Fill the rest of the jar, to the top, with your carrier oil (you can even do a combination of oils if you like. In all of my salves, I steep my herbs in a combination of extra virgin olive oil and extra virgin coconut oil) and cover with a lid. Set out in the sun or a sunny window and give a good shake to the jar ever day for 2 weeks. Using a cheese cloth lined strainer, strain the oil from your herbs and squeeze out any remaining oil to get the most of the oil as possible.

Oven Infusion Method

When I don't have sunshine out here in Texas, this is the method I like to use the most. I find it the easiest to leave it be without having to refill water in the bottom of a double boiler like the stove-top method. Turn your oven on the lowest setting that you can. I like to use a 1/2 gallon mason jar but this can be done in smaller. Fill your jar 1/4-1/2 full of your herbs and cover with oil to the top and cover with a lid. Set the mason jar on its side on a cookie sheet (I use one with a rim so that any oil that might leak out from the lid won't fall onto my oven's heating element) and put in the oven on the middle rack. Every couple of hours pull jar out of the oven and give 2 or 3 shakes. Leave in the oven for 24-48 hours. Using a cheese cloth lined strainer, strain the oil from your herbs and squeeze out any remaining oil to get the most of the oil as possible.

Stove top Infusion Method

This is a good quick method if you don't have the time to wait 2 weeks for a solar infusion to complete. In a double boiler drop in 1/4 part herbs to 1 part oil and allow to steep over the heat for several hours. I see people saying to leave it overnight, but there is no way to do that with a double boiler. Only do this if you are using a crock pot (which you can also use instead of the stove). Using a cheese cloth lined strainer, strain the oil from your herbs and squeeze out any remaining oil to get the most of the oil as possible.

Magic Healing Oil

I use this herbal infused oil in all kinds of salves, body butters, lip balms, bum sprays, and more! You can substitute the Magic Healing Oil into the baby butt balm, bohemi' mama's boobie balm, calendula antiseptic owie cream, shaving cream, or any other recipe that calls for a liquid oil in it. This oil is filled with skin healing herbs that help to minimize and reduce scarring and stretch marks by stimulating the production of collagen at the site of wounds.

INGREDEINTS

- 1 part calendula
- 1 part comfrey
- 1 part st. john's wort
- 1 part plantain
- extra virgin olive oil

Anti-Inflammatory Oil

Arnica is a flowering herb with a longstanding history in relieving muscle pain, bruises, and arthritis. One of the best anti-inflammatory herbs to use in sports medicine, arnica works the best if applied immediately after the injury, externally in a cream or salve. My version of arnica oil is ramped up with other anti-inflammatory herbs that are also known to be antispasmodic, and analgesic. This oil can be used on it's own as a fantastic massage oil, or it can be used in the Sore Muscles Salve and Aunt Flo's Soothing Salve.

INGREDEINTS

- 2 parts arnica
- 1 part st. john's wort
- 1 part chamomile
- 1 part peppermint leaf
- 1 part willow bark
- extra virgin olive oil

Anti-Fungal Oil

There are many herbs that are very helpful to healing a fungal infection, but the two that are most notable and usually can be found in the best of herbal anti-fungal salves are chaparral and black walnut. This Anti-Fungal Oil can be used alone as an oil or added to the Fungus Amungus Anti-Fungal Salve.

INGREDEINTS

- 2 parts chaparral

- 2 parts black walnut hulls
- 1 part echinacea
- 1 part calendula
- extra virgin olive oil

Herbal Infused Vinegars

Herbal infused vinegars have been used since the dawn of time. Early Gypsies formulated many healing herbal infused vinegars, and they used them in everything from hair conditioning rinses, antiseptic mouthwashes, headache remedies, soothing aftershaves, foot baths, and more! Making an herbal infused vinegar is extremely easy, and they can be used in all sorts of recipes! Combine herbs to fill a wide-mouthed, glass mason jar. Fill jar, so that the herbs are completely covered, with raw unfiltered apple cider vinegar. Cover tightly and put in a warm sunny location for 2 to 3 weeks. Shake the jar once a day to mix things up evenly. Strain herbs from liquid and store in the fridge for a really long shelf-life. The uses with these herbal infused vinegars, are endless.

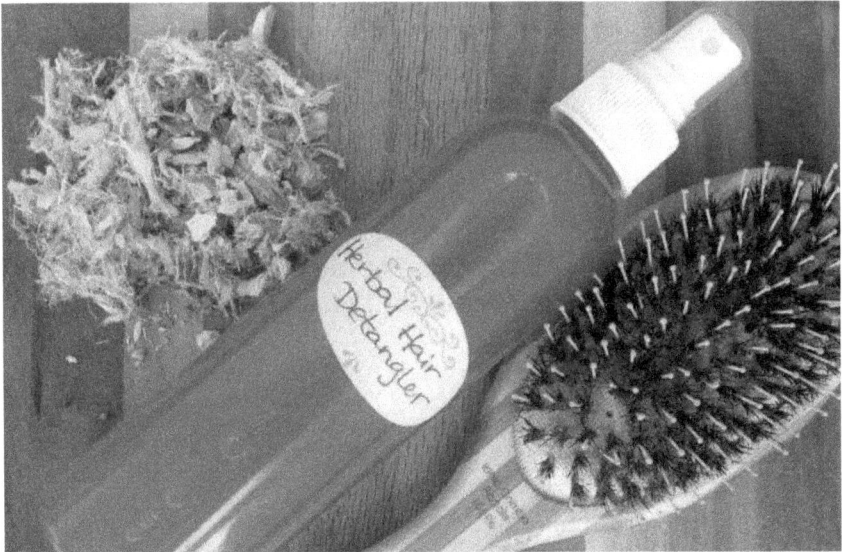

Silken Goddess Hair Apple Cider Vinegar

I use this herbal infused vinegar in everything hair related. I can't get enough of it! Marshmallow root is a mucilage giving herb that gives any hair recipe that conditioning "slip" that helps to detangle and condition your hair. The combination of hair healing herbs in this recipe helps with hair growth, thickness, and even repairing damaged hair. I use this infusion in my apple cider vinegar hair rinse, detangling spray, and all of my no-poo recipes for healthy hippy hair.

INGREDEINTS

- 2 parts marshmallow root
- 1 part horsetail
- 1 part lavender
- 1 part oatstraw
- 1 part rosemary
- raw unfiltered apple cider vinegar

Vinegar of the Thieves

Vinegar of the Thieves originated sometime around the 15th century, when the bubonic plague was running rampant through Europe and Asia. Four thieves from Europe, who were notoriously robbing the infectious dead bodies of all their possessions, miraculously never contracted the highly infectious plague. This led to deep inquiry in court after they were finely caught and charged with theft. The magistrate offered them a deal, their secret for a reduced sentence. Taking the deal, they told stories of their knowledge of herbs and their abilities to keep themselves germ free by using antiviral herbs infused in vinegar and burning antiviral herbs all around them.

This vinegar infusion is based upon this story. With it's antibacterial and antiviral properties, this vinegar can be used full strength to clean the house and kill germs or diluted and sprayed on yourself to repel insects. This is a really mighty insect repellent! This spray is safe to be used on your whole family, pet's included!

INGREDEINTS

- 1 part rosemary
- 1 part lavender
- 1 part peppermint
- ¼ part cloves
- 1 part sage
- 1 stick of cinnamon
- raw unfiltered apple cider vinegar

www.ingramcontent.com/pod-product-compliance
Lightning Source LLC
Chambersburg PA
CBHW031209270326
41931CB00006B/485